*Clinical Supervision in
Occupational Therapy*

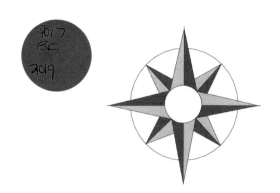

Clinical

A GUIDE

Supervision in

FOR FIELDWORK

Occupational

AND PRACTICE

Therapy

Donna M. Costa, MS, OTR/L

Foreword by Susan K. Meyers, EdD, MBA, OTR, FAOTA

AOTA
PRESS®

The American
Occupational Therapy
Association, Inc.

Vision Statement
AOTA advances occupational therapy as the pre-eminent profession in promoting the health, productivity, and quality of life of individuals and society through the therapeutic application of occupation.

Mission Statement
The American Occupational Therapy Association advances the quality, availability, use, and support of occupational therapy through standard-setting, advocacy, education, and research on behalf of its members and the public.

AOTA Staff
Frederick P. Somers, *Executive Director*
Christopher M. Bluhm, *Chief Operating Officer*
Audrey Rothstein, *Director, Marketing and Communications*

Chris Davis, *Managing Editor, AOTA Press*
Timothy Sniffin, *Production Editor*
Carrie Mercadante, *Editorial Assistant*

Robert A. Sacheli, *Manager, Creative Services*
Sarah E. Ely, *Book Production Coordinator*

Marge Wasson, *Marketing Manager*
Stephanie Heishman, *Marketing Specialist*
John Prudente, *Marketing Specialist*

The American Occupational Therapy Association, Inc.
4720 Montgomery Lane
Bethesda, MD 20814
Phone: 301-652-AOTA (2682)
TDD: 800-377-8555
Fax: 301-652-7711
www.aota.org
To order: 1-877-404-AOTA (2682)
© 2007 by the American Occupational Therapy Association, Inc.

Disclaimers
This publication is designed to provide accurate and authoritative information in regard to the subject matter covered. It is sold or distributed with the understanding that the publisher is not engaged in rendering legal, accounting, or other professional service. If legal advice or other expert assistance is required, the services of a competent professional person should be sought.
—*From the Declaration of Principles jointly adopted by the American Bar Association and a Committee of Publishers and Associations*

It is the objective of the American Occupational Therapy Association to be a forum for free expression and interchange of ideas. The opinions expressed by the contributors to this work are their own and not necessarily those of the American Occupational Therapy Association.

ISBN 10: 1-56900-218-5
ISBN 13: 978-1-56900-218-6

Library of Congress Control Number: 2007925093

Design by Sarah E. Ely
Composition by Electronic Quill Publishing Services, Silver Spring, MD
Printed by Automated Graphics, Inc., White Plains, MD

Citation: Costa, D. (2007). *Clinical supervision in occupational therapy: A guide for fieldwork and practice.* Bethesda, MD: AOTA Press.

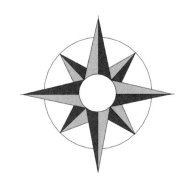

Contents

Foreword

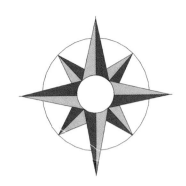

Most students believe clinical education will be the defining experience in their transition to becoming occupational therapists. We all have had clinical education experiences, some exemplary and others nearly unbearable, but whether good or bad, they taught us, among other things, how to be a clinical supervisor. As this book illustrates, however, this significant portion of education is entrusted to those who have no idea how to be an effective clinical supervisor. Learning to be a therapist does not prepare us to teach future therapists or supervise others in clinical practice, both skills necessary to becoming a good clinical supervisor.

Years ago, I examined occupational therapy clinical education and found that, while some fieldwork supervisors took the responsibility of preparing future clinicians seriously and as a responsibility to ensure competent future practice of the profession, others quite disliked the task assigned to them. It was no surprise to discover that students who had the responsible supervisor had more positive learning experiences than those who had the misfortune of being assigned to the unwilling supervisor. Both types of supervisors, however, constructed student fieldwork experiences based on their skills and knowledge of being therapists and less on principles of adult learning and theories of supervision.

This book provides therapists who, either voluntarily or by assignment, become clinical supervisors with information that will prepare them to provide students with important professional learning experiences in practice. Providing clinical supervision is a courageous activity in which the supervisor must inform and make demands of students in applying classroom skills and knowledge as well as professional behaviors. The supervisor needs to be confident in his or her abilities to make these demands and to take risks to try new methods that reflect changes in learners and environments that challenge even the best clinicians.

All who have supervised students or studied clinical education and believe in a strong future for our profession will appreciate what this book offers. The role of clinical supervision is one that should not be left to chance; it is too important and deserves to be more uniformly approached based on theoretical and practical knowledge. To those who read this book and apply what you learn to supervise future therapists, thank you. You are the shapers of our professional future.

—*Susan K. Meyers, EdD, MBA, OTR, FAOTA*
University of Indianapolis

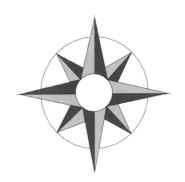

Preface

Readers familiar with the book *Charlotte's Web* by E. B. White (1952) may recall a conversation between Charlotte, the spider, and Wilbur, the pig. Charlotte, who just has finished spinning her egg sac containing 514 spider babies, tells Wilbur that it is "my magnum opus, my great work, the finest thing I have ever made" (p. 144). That is what this book is for me. I have been an occupational therapist for the majority of my life and have supervised fieldwork students throughout my career. Like most practitioners, I learned how to supervise students by trial and error, discovering what works and what does not through my successes and failures.

Fieldwork education is critical to professional education; it links education and practice and is an extension of the occupational therapy curriculum. And yet, despite its importance, fieldwork education has remained relatively untouched by research, theory development, or training. Today's students are tomorrow's occupational therapists and occupational therapy assistants, and the fastest way to influence practice is through students. Students are receiving the benefits of cutting-edge research and theory development in the classroom. Their fieldwork educators, however, often do not have access to the most recent literature, research, or emerging trends on clinical supervision.

As in professions such as social work, psychology, counseling, nursing, and physical therapy, attempts are being made increasingly to elevate the practice of fieldwork education by making a commitment to train those who direct this critical piece of professional education. In the field of clinical supervision, a growing body of knowledge is becoming available to guide the practice of supervision. Clinical supervision is developing as an intervention in its own right, with a distinct body of knowledge and theories and an increasing evidence base.

Our colleagues in other health professions such as physical therapy and speech–language pathology have grappled with some of the same issues we face. In her 1951 article on physical therapy clinical instruction, Beatrice Whitcomb stated,

> In any educational program the most important single factor for
> success is the instructor. The satisfaction and effectiveness of the
> students in their clinical practice experience, as well as many of
> their future attitudes toward their work, will be depend almost
> entirely upon the quality of supervision. In addition to a broad
> knowledge of the subject and certain personal traits, it is essential

that the teaching supervisor have a liking for and a degree of skill in teaching. (p. 129)

Similarly, physical therapist Joy Higgs and speech pathologist Lindy McAllister have stated,

> A great deal of the success of clinical education rests on the shoulders of clinical educators, their own abilities and personal attributes, and the preparation and support they receive. The lack of adequate preparation of clinical educators is a chronic problem in the health sciences. As a result, clinical educators lack an explicit theoretical and philosophical framework for their educational activities, myths about clinical education are pervasive, integration of academic and clinical curricula suffers, and there is a mismatch between the theory and practice of clinical education. (p. 156)

Several influential writers in occupational therapy have commented on the lack of support and training for fieldwork educators. Cohn and Frum (1988) noted that, despite the importance of fieldwork and the demands placed on fieldwork educators, training largely has been absent: "Lack of experience and absence of training frequently leave the new supervisor searching for direction. More often than not the process of being an effective fieldwork educator is an evolutionary one based on trial and error" (p. 325). This state of affairs is not unique to occupational therapy in the United States; our colleagues in the United Kingdom are facing similar issues: "It is surprising that the pivotal and complex role of the clinician as supervisor has received scant attention in the literature. This paucity of information stems from an assumption (which permeates the literature on supervision) that expertise as a clinician implies expertise as a supervisor. However, there is no empirical evidence to support this implication" (Sweeney, Webley, & Treacher, 2001a, p. 337).

This book attempts to address the gaps in the occupational therapy knowledge base on the theory and practice of clinical supervision. In this volume, I have attempted to provide a theoretical and philosophical framework for clinical supervision, to correct myths about it, and to bridge the connection between the theory and practice of clinical education and supervision.

Some readers may question my use of the term *clinical supervision* instead of *clinical education* or *fieldwork education*. Across the health professions, *clinical education* is used to describe the placement of students in clinical practice settings, where they learn to apply the knowledge gained in the classroom and construct new knowledge. In occupational therapy, the practice of clinical education is called *fieldwork education* and the people who provide this intervention are *fieldwork educators*. A conscious shift has been made in the profession away from the use of *fieldwork supervisor* in favor of the term *fieldwork educator* in recognition of the active learning process inherent in fieldwork. As I discuss in Chapter 2, however, the term *clinical supervision,* first used in the early 1900s, came from the social work profession. Alfred Kadushin (1976, 1992), an influential writer in social work clinical supervision, reinforced some of the original writings of John Dawson, who in 1926 originally described the three functions of supervision as administrative, educational, and supportive. I propose that all clinical supervision has these three functions. In fieldwork, the intervention is mainly educational. In clinical supervision between peers, the supportive function is emphasized. In running a department, the administrative function takes the foreground.

The *International Classification of Functioning, Disability, and Health (ICF;* World Health Organization, 2001) was in part the result of a vigorous attempt to persuade health care professionals to speak a common language. To be consistent with the language of the *ICF,* the third edition of the *Uniform Terminology for Occupational Therapy* (American Occupational Therapy Association [AOTA], 1994) was rescinded and replaced by the *Occupational Therapy Practice Framework: Domain and Process* (AOTA, 2002c). Effective interdisciplinary collaboration is not possible if health care professionals do not speak a common language. So I propose that in fieldwork education, occupational therapists and occupational therapy assistants use the terms *fieldwork educators* and *clinical supervision.*

Across practice settings, occupational therapy practitioners at all levels seek out and receive clinical supervision from colleagues who assist them in continuing their lifelong learning through advanced study, clinical reasoning activities, evidence-based practice, and reflective practice. In managing occupational therapy departments, department heads use clinical supervision to drive excellence in the workplace, promote the use of evidence-based practice, and increase accountability for patient care. Clinical supervision is, therefore, a specific practice or intervention and has a clearly delineated theoretical base.

This book will be useful for occupational therapist and occupational therapy assistant students who are preparing for their Level II fieldwork experience and want to be proactive in engaging in a more student-centered, active learning experience. It will be very helpful to new or novice occupational therapy practitioners who are on that steep learning curve of the first few years of practice; it will assist them in identifying the body of knowledge in the area of clinical supervision that they were probably not exposed to in school. For fieldwork educators, regardless of their number of years of experience, this book is essential reading. To provide effective clinical supervision to fieldwork students, one must know what it is, be able to self-assess one's knowledge and skills, and create a professional development plan that addresses the further refinement of those skills.

For occupational therapy practitioners at all levels, this book fills a void in the literature on the theory and practice of clinical supervision. Many professions, including occupational therapy, espouse clinical supervision as a way to gain clinical reasoning skills and acquire advanced practice knowledge from a more senior practitioner. Lastly, for managers of practice settings, who use all three functions of clinical supervision—administrative, supportive, and educational—this book provides a theoretical base for the practice of clinical supervision.

—*Donna M. Costa, MS, OTR/L*

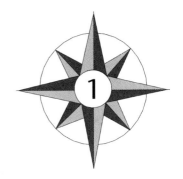

What Is Clinical Supervision?

Like guides, we walk ahead of our students, at times beside them, and at times we follow their lead. In sensing where to walk lies our art. For as we support [them] in their struggle, challenge them toward their best, and cast light on their path ahead, we do so in the name of our respect for their potential and our care for their growth.

(Daloz, 1999, p. 244)

Occupational therapists and occupational therapy assistants spend years of extensive training in the classroom to learn the theory and practice of occupational therapy with numerous populations and in varied practice settings. In fieldwork, they learn to apply this extensive body of knowledge, making fieldwork the bridge between the classroom and the clinic. The transition from student to practitioner is facilitated by more senior occupational therapists and occupational therapy assistants, who guide, teach, and provide feedback to students and ensure that quality services are provided to their clients. This process of facilitation is referred to as *clinical supervision,* which includes not only fieldwork education but also guidance throughout the process of lifelong learning that frames occupational therapists' professional development.

The Hippocratic Oath dates back to 400 BC and alludes to the process of clinical supervision:

> I swear by Apollo the physician, and Aesculapius, and Health, and All-Heal, and all the gods and goddesses, that according to my ability and judgment, I will keep this oath and this stipulation to reckon him who taught me this Art equally dear to me as my parents, to share my substance with him, and relieve his necessities if required; to look upon his offspring in the same footing as my own brothers . . . . (cited in Bernard & Goodyear, 2004,[*] p. 2)

This ancient oath underscores the value of more senior members of a profession watching over and guiding more junior members and serving as gatekeepers for that profession. Clinical supervision is the process of linking formal theory taught in the classroom with real-world practice. Professors test students' competencies in the classroom through questions, examinations, practical lab exams, and written and oral assignments. Clinical supervisors test students' competencies in the clinic by watching the treatments they provide clients, providing written and verbal feedback, asking questions, and guiding the development of students' professional behavior.

---

[*] From Bernard, Janine M. & Rodney K. Goodyear, *Fundamentals of Clinical Supervision,* 3rd Edition, published by Allyn & Bacon, Boston. Copyright © 2004 by Pearson Education. Reprinted/adapted by permission of the publisher.

Clinical supervision is therefore a blend of teaching, counseling, evaluation, and consultation, but it is distinct from all of them. Thus, an occupational therapist's or occupational therapy assistant's knowledge and skills as a therapist, teacher, counselor, or consultant not necessarily ensure a positive outcome in providing clinical supervision, because clinical supervision is an intervention in and of itself. Many professionals from many health-related disciplines believe that if they are good practitioners, they will be good supervisors. But, as I will emphasize throughout this book, the skills required of practitioners do not carry over to the realm of clinical supervision.

I once went into a large bookstore and asked for assistance at the service desk. Could they help me find a book on "supervision"? Did I mean "super vision," they asked? At the time, I thought their question absurd, but reflecting on it, supervision is sometimes super vision in that it refers to a clarity of thought and perception about another person. A good supervisor has a type of crystal ball that permits him or her to look deep into the student and see beyond the façade to see what is driving him or her to act in a particular way. All occupational therapists and occupational therapy assistants have had clients who made them wonder how to proceed next. Indeed, the experience of looking back on a situation after the fact and identifying a much better solution—sometimes referred to as the "Monday-morning quarterback syndrome"—is a normal phenomenon of professional life. A competent clinical supervisor, however, is able to examine the situation objectively in the moment and provide timely advice.

Definitions of Clinical Supervision

Supervision is defined in the dictionary as "the action, process, or occupation of supervising: a critical watching and directing (as of activities or a course of action)" (*Merriam-Webster's New Collegiate Dictionary,* 2003, p. 1255). The word has its etymological roots in the Latin words *super,* meaning "over," and *videre,* meaning "to see more at WIT" (p. 1170). *Wit* is defined as "mental capability and resourcefulness, astuteness of perception or judgment, the ability to relate seemingly disparate things so as to illuminate. . ." (p. 1348). In these root definitions are most of the elements of supervision. The allied health literature has offered some more specific definitions of clinical supervision.

Psychologists Carol Loganbill, Emily Hardy, and Ursula Delworth (1982) defined *clinical supervision* as "an intensive, interpersonally focused one-to-one relationship in which one person is designated to facilitate the development of therapeutic competence in the other person" (p. 4). This definition was used in an earlier publication of the American Occupational Therapy Association (AOTA; Frum & Opacich, 1987), and it was one of the first formal definitions of clinical supervision that emphasized a developmental orientation. This definition, however, omits group and collaborative models of supervision, and it mentions only briefly the therapeutic competence of the supervisee. There is no mention of the client or the practice setting. It also connotes a hierarchical relationship that places one person over another rather than recognizing the cooperative and collaborative aspects of learning together. Frum and Opacich rephrased Loganbill and colleagues' definition as follows:

> Supervision is regarded as an association, an alliance between two people. The relationship is of such importance that it has the potential to increase the capabilities of another person. Our model particularly refers to increasing the abilities of another in the professional role of the therapist. (p. 3)

The 1991 AOTA publication *Self-Paced Instruction for Clinical Education and Supervision* (SPICES) defined supervision as "a process in which two or more people participate in a joint effort to promote, establish, maintain, and/or elevate a level of performance or service" (p. 815). This definition acknowledges that the clinical supervision process may be with more than one supervisee and addressed the collaborative aspect of clinical supervision. The welfare and safety of the client, however, are not addressed, nor is there any mention of the practice setting. That same publication also offered the following definition of supervision:

> A mutual undertaking between the supervisor and supervisee that fosters growth and development; ensures appropriate utilization of training and potential; encourages creativity and innovation; and provides guidance, support, encouragement and respect while working towards the goals of the facility. (p. 815)

This definition expands on several qualities inherent in clinical supervision, including the interpersonal aspects of working with a supervisee, and it includes the practice setting. The client is left out of this equation, however, and there is no suggestion of a developmental progression.

Loretta J. Bradley (1989), an educational psychologist, put forth another definition of clinical supervision as "facilitating personal and professional development, improving competencies and promoting accountability in service and programs" (p. 26). This definition added the issue of personal development that had not yet been addressed directly. It failed, however, to include the protection of the client, and it did not address the practice setting.

Psychology researcher Allen K. Hess (1980) provided still another definition of clinical supervision as "a quintessential interpersonal interaction with the general goal that one person, the supervisor, meets with another, the supervisee, in an effort to make the latter more effective in helping people" (p. 25). This definition is similar to Loganbill and colleagues,' with its focus on the individual aspect of supervision, but again it does not mention the practice setting or the client.

Social worker Alfred Kadushin (1976) wrote extensively on the role of clinical supervision in social work, and his definition encompassed the three functions that he viewed as inherent in supervision: educational, administrative, and supportive. He defined supervision as

> an administrative and clinical process designed to facilitate the counselor's ability to deliver the best possible service to clients, both quantitative and qualitative, in accordance with agency policy, procedures, and the context of a positive relationship between counselor and supervisor. (p. 20)

What is different about Kadushin's definition is the inclusion of the supportive role of supervision, or what he referred to as the

> expressive–supportive leadership function of supervision. The supervisor has the responsibility of sustaining worker morale, helping with job-related discouragements and discontents, and giving supervisees a sense of worth as professionals, a sense of belonging in the agency, and a sense of security in their performance. (p. 19)

This concept is particularly relevant for clinical supervision as a professional development activity that provides the occupational therapy practitioner with opportunities for lifelong learning.

David Powell (1993), an internationally recognized leader in clinical supervision whose work was targeted mainly toward those working in the addictions field, developed the concept of *blended supervision,* which he defined as "a disciplined, tutorial process wherein principles are transformed into practical skills, with four overlapping foci: administrative, evaluative, clinical, and supportive" (p. 9). This definition built on Kadushin's (1976) concept of clinical supervision as having multiple foci and framed it in a developmental construct. As with many other definitions, however, it omitted protection of the client's welfare.

One definition that emphasized the issue of monitoring client's welfare was put forth by psychologist Robert Haynes, human services professor Gerald Corey, and psychologist and counselor Patrice Moulton (2003):

> Clinical supervision is best defined as a process whereby consistent observation and evaluation of the counseling process is provided by a trained and experienced professional who recognizes and is competent in the unique body of knowledge and skill required for professional development. It should be noted that clinical supervision is also defined by many external forces,

including governing bodies, licensing agencies, and the settings in which we work. (p. 3)

The other unique feature of this definition is the notion that the supervisor has certain competencies in supervision, referred to in the definition as a "unique body of knowledge and skills." Unfortunately, this definition is limited by its reference to the counseling process.

Psychologist Jane M. Campbell's (2006) definition of clinical supervision differentiated it from counseling and therapy:

> The primary purpose of clinical supervision is to review practitioners' work to increase their skills and help them solve problems in order to provide clients the optimal quality of service possible and prevent any harm from occurring. Therefore, it is a teaching and training role as well as a monitoring function. What sets clinical supervision aside from the other types of relationships, such as psychotherapy or consultation, is the presence of an evaluative component. Another important but frequently overlooked variable that needs to be considered is the fact that clinical supervision, for the majority of supervisees, is not voluntary. This evaluative component, along with the non-voluntary nature of supervision, cast issues of power, trust, safety, and control into the center of the clinical supervisees experience and the supervisory relationship. (p. 2)

Although this definition addressed the issue of monitoring client's welfare, it also suggested some other issues that require knowledge and skills on the part of the supervisor.

Educational and professional development researcher Della Fish and lecturer Sheila Twinn (1997) emphasized the learning component in clinical supervision and the requirement that clinical educators have an awareness of the process of learning:

> Quality supervision involves a detailed understanding and appreciation of how we learn new practice and therefore how the learner can be supported in doing so. [Clinical] educators should not just be content experts. They should also act as facilitators assisting students to learn from themselves by reflecting on experiences. (p. 39)

Psychologists Carol Falendar and Edward Shafranske (2004) recently provided one of the most comprehensive definitions of supervision:

> Supervision is a distinct professional activity in which education and training aimed at developing science-informed practice are facilitated through a collaborative interpersonal process. It

involves observation, evaluation, feedback, the facilitation of supervisee self-assessment, and the acquisition of knowledge and skills by instruction, modeling, and mutual problem solving. In addition, by building on the recognition of the strengths and talents of the supervisee, supervision encourages self-efficacy. Supervision ensures that clinical consultation is conducted in a competent manner in which ethical standards, legal prescriptions, and professional practices are used to promote and protect the welfare of the client, the profession, and society at large. (p. 3)

This definition includes the monitoring of client welfare but also addresses the professional development of the supervisee in a collaborative relationship. It further discusses the need for evidence-based practice—with clients as well as in supervision contexts.

Best Definition of Clinical Supervision

The definition of clinical supervision that appears to have all of the necessary elements was developed by education and counseling professor Janine M. Bernard and psychologist and professor Rodney K. Goodyear (2004):

Supervision is an intervention provided by a more senior member of the profession to a more junior member of that same profession. This relationship is evaluative, extends over time, and has the simultaneous purposes of enhancing the professional functioning of the more junior person(s), monitoring the quality of professional services offered to the clients that he, she, or they see, and serving as a gatekeeper for those who are about to enter that particular profession. (p. 6)

In the following paragraphs, I examine each element of this definition as it relates to occupational therapy practice.

"Supervision is an intervention." Although supervision is sometimes like therapy, sometimes like coaching, sometimes like teaching, and sometimes like consultation, it is really a blend of all of these elements. More importantly, supervision is a separate intervention in its own right. As such, it has specific competencies and a specific body of knowledge that has been growing slowly but to date includes only limited outcomes research. The challenge facing practitioners from all disciplines is to delineate this body of knowledge into distinct approaches and then study the efficacy of one approach over another with different practitioners in different practice settings. Only then can one answer the question "What works best with whom in what setting?"

"Provided by a more senior member of a profession to a more junior member of that same profession." In fieldwork, there is a fieldwork educator and a student.

In Level II fieldwork, the clinical educator must be an occupational therapist or occupational therapy assistant with at least 1 year of experience. Occupational therapists can supervise either occupational therapy students or occupational therapy assistant students, while occupational therapy assistants may supervise only occupational therapy assistant students. "Senior" does not imply age but a recognition of more professional experience. So there is a hierarchical relationship between a more senior and a more junior member of the occupational therapy profession. But this part of the definition also would apply to clinical supervision outside of fieldwork. Occupational therapy students are introduced to the concept of lifelong learning. Certainly, some of this learning comes from attending conferences and other continuing education events. But the current health care climate demands accountability and provision of continuous quality improvement, which ongoing clinical supervision can provide.

Most occupational therapists and occupational therapy assistants have a designated supervisor, who may be a department head or the owner of a company. It may be the person with the authority to countersign clinical notes or other documentation. Some occupational therapy managers meet with their supervisees regularly to review caseloads or provide annual performance evaluations. Other managers' supervisory roles may be purely administrative, with minimal time available to discuss clinical issues. For practitioners whose supervisors have little time to provide clinical supervision, there are other ways to obtain meaningful supervision. Increasingly, occupational therapy practitioners are finding mentors who can guide their lifelong learning and provide them with feedback and direction. Peer supervision is another vehicle; occupational therapists and occupational therapy assistants can form groups to review cases, learn new techniques, and receive feedback.

"The relationship is evaluative." Evaluation is an important element of clinical supervision, especially in fieldwork education. Fieldwork educators complete the *Fieldwork Performance Evaluation* (AOTA, 2002a, 2002b) at midterm and at the end of the fieldwork assignment for each supervisee. There is some form of evaluation following a Level I fieldwork assignment, often focused on providing feedback to the student on his or her demonstration (or lack thereof) of professional behaviors and emerging clinical skills. Throughout the fieldwork experience, the effective fieldwork educator continuously provides students with either written or verbal feedback and evaluates their performance and competency in evaluation, treatment, documentation, and professional behaviors. Sometimes this feedback is formal, involving a weekly written report that summarizes what the student has learned during the past week and sets up learning goals for the following week. Sometimes the feedback is informal and verbal, perhaps given during the break following a meeting or treatment session.

In clinical supervision outside of fieldwork, the function remains evaluative. A supervisor asks a supervisee questions such as "Why did you provide that treatment to that client?" or "Let's review the treatment course for Mrs. X so we know where we went wrong and how to avoid this situation in the future." In some health care facilities, the manager's role is to provide both clinical and administrative oversight to employees. This oversight might take the form of grand rounds–type presentations in which the supervisee formally presents a case or a treatment and has opportunities to ask questions and receive feedback. Or the department may have monthly in-service presentations to keep therapists current in emerging technologies.

In one of my first jobs as an occupational therapist, in a county hospital's psychiatric service, every member of the treatment team had an individual supervisor who spent a minimum of 1 hour per week in a one-on-one session, reviewing cases and treatment provided. My supervisor was very analytical and preferred viewing videotapes of my treatment groups. So each week, we watched a tape from a group session I had led the previous week, and we discussed my responses. Although the scrutiny was painful at the time, this was a tremendous opportunity to receive feedback from a more seasoned clinician on the style, timing, and intent of my interventions with clients. I learned a great deal about running groups from these supervisory sessions, although I did not particularly enjoy the videotaping.

"This relationship . . . extends over time" and thus has a developmental aspect. Supervisees come to fieldwork as neophytes, often unsure of themselves but usually eager to learn. The supervision provided on the first day of their fieldwork experience is not the same as that provided at the end of their Level II fieldwork experience. Supervision changes as students change, just as treatment changes during the course of work with a client in response to his or her needs. So there is not only a developmental aspect to clinical supervision but also a graded response. Standard 10.0 of the Accreditation Council for Occupational Therapy Education (ACOTE, 2007) states that supervision "must be initially direct and then may be decreased to less direct supervision as is appropriate for the setting, the client's needs, and the ability of the student" (p. 43).

"This relationship . . . has the simultaneous purposes of enhancing the professional functioning of the more junior person(s)." Professional functioning is best achieved through observation and role modeling by the supervisor. Role modeling is an inherent function in clinical supervision; if supervisees are to demonstrate professional behavior, then supervisors must model this behavior. Supervisors progressively enhance the professional functioning of their supervisees by promoting clinical reasoning and reflective practice and by guiding personal and professional growth.

". . . of monitoring the quality of professional services offered to the client that she, he, or they see. . . ." This aspect of clinical supervision has an inherent legal and ethical component. A supervisor's job is to ensure that clients receive the

highest quality services that they are entitled to. The supervisor's cosignature on a supervisee's documentation implies that the supervisor has observed and concurs with the supervisee's treatment recommendations. *Vicarious liability* refers to the supervisor's liability for any untoward action by the supervisee that harms the client. If and when a supervisor sees harm being done to a client, he or she is legally bound to confront the supervisee and step in to correct the situation. Extreme situations may lead a supervisor to terminate the supervisee's fieldwork or even employment.

". . . and serving as a gatekeeper for those who are about to enter that particular profession." The gatekeeper function often causes supervisors great anxiety, particularly in cases in which they have to terminate fieldwork for a particular student or give him or her a failing grade. Although no one enjoys terminating or failing a student, it is a professional responsibility to ensure that occupational therapy professionals conform to the spirit and intent of the profession. Serving as a gatekeeper for occupational therapy means allowing only those students who have demonstrated entry-level competency in a particular practice setting to pass fieldwork. Students may achieve high marks in the classroom, but unless they are able to apply that knowledge, they cannot and should not be admitted into the academy of occupational therapists and occupational therapy assistants. Academic grades rarely predict clinical performance, and students must successfully complete both their academic course of study and their fieldwork to become certified or licensed.

Developing One's Own Definition of Supervision

The definitions discussed in this chapter offer a framework for supervisors to develop a personal definition of supervision in line with their own frames of reference and personal and professional identities. One way to begin to define clinical supervision is to think of metaphors that describe the supervisory process. Proctor (1991), for example, examined the process of supervision as a metaphoric expression of the supervisor's prior life experiences:

> A number of my colleagues asked me what type of archetypes went into taking the trainer role; we immediately identified a number. These are Guru, or Wise Woman, from which wisdom is expected, and the Earth Mother—the all-provider, unconditional positive regarder. In contrast, there is the Clown or Jester— enjoying performance, and cloaking his truth in riddles, without taking any responsibility for how it is received. The Patriarch creates order and unselfconsciously wields power. The Actor/Director allocates roles and tasks and holds the Drama; the Bureaucrat demands compliance to the letter of the law. The Whore gives services for money, which can be indistinguishable

from love, and re-engages with group after group. There is even the Warrior—valiant for truth; and of course the Judge— upholding standards and impartially assessing. The Shepherd/ Sheep dog gently and firmly rounds up and pens. (p. 65)

Page and Wosket (1994) likened their definition of clinical supervision to the process of riding a bicycle:

There are many different types of two-wheel cycles, some different because they are designed and made by different manufacturers who give priority to a particular quality in their product. We could liken counselor supervision to the tandem [bicycle]—having two riders rather than the usual one offers a means whereby the inexperienced rider might coach an inexperienced one in the saddle. (pp. 3–4)

Hillerbrand (1989) used the metaphor of parents teaching their children life skills in describing supervision in the context of psychologist Liv Vygotsky's theories of learning (1962, 1978):

Vygotsky proposed that cognitive skills are acquired through social interaction. Unskilled persons learn cognitive skills by assuming more and more responsibility from experts during performance (what he called "expert scaffolding"). Novices first observe an expert's cognitive activity while the experts do most of the work. As novices begin to perform the skills, they receive feedback from the experts on their performance; as they learn to perform the skill correctly, they begin to assume more responsibility for the cognitive skill. Finally, novices assume the major responsibility for the cognitive skill, and experts become passive observers. (p. 294)

Still another analogy is drawn from the parenting literature, borrowing from Winnicott's description of the "good-enough mother"—the mother who is able to tolerate the mischievous behavior of her child without overreacting because she does not view it as a personal attack. Hawkins and Shohet (2000) used an analogy for supervision in which

the "good-enough" counselor, psychotherapist, or other helping professional can survive the negative attacks of the client through the strength of being held within and by the supervisory relationship. We have often seen very competent workers reduced to severe doubts about themselves and their abilities to function in the work through absorbing disturbance from clients. The supervisor's role is not just to reassure the worker, but to allow the

emotional disturbance to be felt within the safer setting of the
supervisory relationship, where it can be survived, reflected upon,
and learned from. Supervision thus provides a container that
holds the helping relationship. (p. 3)

This chapter has attempted to summarize some of the many definitions of clinical supervision that have appeared in professional literature. Occupational therapy practitioners need to collaborate with professionals and scholars from other disciplines. To be effective at doing so, practitioners need to speak a common language and contribute to the collaborative building of knowledge.

 ## Learning Activities

1. Having read the section on using metaphors and analogies to describe clinical supervision, create your own metaphors that describe your experience of clinical supervision.

2. Many definitions of clinical supervision have been offered in this chapter; some of the concepts will resonate with you more deeply than others. Take a few minutes to think about your practice setting, and come up with your own definition of clinical supervision.

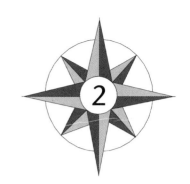

History of Clinical Supervision

This chapter explores the history of clinical supervision, beginning with the fields of medicine and social work and examining its development in occupational therapy fieldwork education. Physicians, as well as other professionals, learned their craft from those who came before them, and practices were passed down from one generation to another in an apprentice model, in which the novice learned skills by performing them under the watchful eye of the master.

Powell (1993) traced the roots of supervision to late-19th-century New England, where masters oversaw the work of artisans. According to Powell, the term *supervision* was used to describe the activities of the person in charge of a work crew. This person, called a "foreman," set the tone and pace for the workers as he chanted "one, two, three, up!" (p. 3).

The Profession of Medicine

In medicine, supervision and consultation can be traced back to the 13th century to the statutes of the Guild of Doctors and Apothecaries of Florence, which required that consultation be sought in difficult patient cases (Kaslow, 1977). During the 15th century in France, physicians attempted to form a professional association and proposed a requirement that its members consult with a senior colleague in "desperate or deadly" patient cases (p. 8). A satirical poem written in 1709 by physician Samuel Garth referred disparagingly to the practice of consultation:

> grave Physicians at a Consult met
> about each Symptom how they disagree
> and how unanimous in case of Fee
> and whilst one Assassin another plies
> with starched civilities,
> the patient dies. (quoted in Kaslow, 1977, pp. 8–9)

With patients from upper socioeconomic classes, consultations took place in the home. Consultation through the mail enabled a patient to avoid a fee: "This was an acceptable practice during the seventeenth and eighteenth centuries, whereby a practitioner would request the opinion of an eminent physician on the basis of a letter describing the case" (Kaslow, 1977, p. 11).

By the late 18th century in the United States, there were about 400 medical school–educated physicians, and they began to form medical associations that encouraged the use of consultation and supervision. The Code of Ethics of the American Medical Association stated in 1847 that "consultations should be promoted in difficult or protracted cases, as they give rise to confidence, energy, and more enlarged views of practice" (quoted in Kaslow, 1977, p. 14). As U.S. medical schools developed in the 19th century, they began to introduce both classroom and clinical instruction:

> At first these schools hired preceptors from among the many physicians experienced in providing such training and, later in the century, from among capable practitioners. As the teaching hospital became an integral part of medical education, there evolved the present system of unremunerated clinical instruction by outstanding practitioners who are rewarded with "hospital privileges" and teaching appointments in conjunction with paid clinical instruction by attending physicians on the hospital staff. (Kutzik, 1977a, p. 18)

The Profession of Social Work

The social work profession has had the most historical influence on the practice of clinical supervision. The profession dates back to the late 19th century, when charity organizations and settlement houses were formed. The primary method of teaching "charity workers," as they were first called, was the apprenticeship approach, defined as "doing in the field under the direction of others who had learned in the same way" (George, 1982, quoted in Caspi & Reid, 2002, p. 32).

The charity organization movement began in Buffalo, New York, in 1878 with the goal of providing financial assistance to families. "Friendly visitors" sent to the homes of families in need were volunteers assigned to provide support and to attempt to influence the behaviors that affected the families' well-being (Kadushin, 1992, p. 2). The work of friendly visitors was supervised by "paid agents," who were early predecessors of what are now called supervisors. The paid agents' caseloads were very high, and turnover was rapid among the volunteer visitors. The New York Association for Improving the Conditions of the Poor was founded in 1843, and it "maintained a paid staff who were to supervise and train volunteers and thus provide continuity of service" (quoted in Kadushin, 1992, p. 3). Paid agents provided friendly visitors with education on methods of interacting with families, consultation on cases, and morale boosting. A manual written in 1901 stated that

> to make friendly visiting succeed, the agents must care to really help the visitor—not merely give what the visitor asks, but with tact and patience what he needs and to go at it simply and informally. The agent must learn patiently how to know and under-

stand the new visitor. Thought must be given to his problems and both direct and indirect means used to help him help himself in working them out with the poor family. (Smith, quoted in Kadushin, 1992, p. 6)

Before the advent of schools of social work, this apprenticeship-like model was the primary mode of learning the craft of the profession. As Burns (1965) described it,

Historically, supervision developed as a way of training staff, paid or volunteer, to do the job at hand. Both supervision and case-work, in the modern sense, developed in the charity organization societies that were established in many United States cities during the last twenty years of the nineteenth century. Numerous volunteer workers were needed to carry out this work of friendly visiting, particularly during periods of economic distress. These volunteer visitors had to be instructed in charity organization principles and methods; their efforts required guidance and coordination; their interest in the work had to be encouraged and sustained. To meet these needs—administrative and educational—supervision was developed. (pp. 785–786)

Kadushin (1976) estimated that by 1890, "78 charity organizations with 174 case workers and 2,017 friendly visitors" existed (p. 5). This system of overseeing the provision of services continued into the early 20th century, when the first schools of social work were developed. From the outset, these schools combined classroom instruction with what was called *field instruction,* a term still used in the social work field.

The first social work text to use the word *supervision* in the title was *Supervision and Education in Charity,* (Brackett, 1904), although this text focused primarily on administrative supervision within charity organizations. The term *supervision* appeared in the social work literature again in 1936 in a work that differentiated between administrative and educational supervision:

The word supervision has become a technical term in social work with a usage not defined in any dictionary. Supervisors in a social agency are responsible for overseeing the job in the generally understood meaning of the word, but they have, in addition, a second function of teaching or training workers under their supervision. . . . Supervision can be defined as an educational process in which a certain equipment of knowledge and skills takes responsibility for training a person with less equipment. (Robinson, 1936, p. 53)

During the 1920s, the popularity of psychoanalytic psychology influenced the training of new social workers, with clinical supervision shifting toward a personal therapy orientation. Clinical supervision increasingly took on an educational role, with an emphasis on analyzing the relationship between the supervisor and supervisee framed by ego psychology theory. It became customary for supervisors to help supervisees resolve their intrapsychic conflicts in the recognition that supervisees could not help others until they were aware of and had resolved their own personal issues:

> The supervisor considers herself a caseworker whose case work
> must embrace not only the student's cases but the student herself.
> This demands, of course, that the supervisor investigate and treat
> the personal problems of the student as the latter investigates and
> treats those of the client. If casework is an art and not merely a
> trade practiced on the handicapped and helpless, it was to be just
> as thoroughly a part of the caseworker's attitude toward herself.
> (Marcus, 1927, quoted in Kadushin, 1992, p. 12)

Clinical supervision was thus seen as a kind of learning alliance between the supervisor and supervisee in which the student therapist learned how to perform therapy while developing his or her own self-awareness in psychoanalytic supervision.

From 1975 on, interest in clinical supervision has increased, and a steadily growing number of texts and journals are published each year describing methods and techniques of supervision. In 1946 Spellman (quoted in Kadushin, 1992) provided a humorous description of the various methods of clinical supervision:

> We've had the "trouble-shooter method": "let me know if
> anything goes wrong and you need me for any emergency—and
> I'll be right there." Then there is the "hit-and-run method": "I'll
> see you in the hall a couple of minutes after the meeting is over
> and we'll check on what happened and what you want for next
> week." Others had worked out the "crutch philosophy": "I'll help
> you get started until you can stand on your own two feet." (p. 15)

The Profession of Occupational Therapy

Early Efforts to Address Student Supervision

Interest in using occupations as curative modalities dates back to the early 20th century, when courses were developed for nurses, social workers, and other hospital workers on the use of arts and crafts. At the Chicago School of Civics and Philanthropy, social reformer and occupational therapy pioneer Julia Lathrop began teaching a 6-week "special course in curative occupations and recreations for attendants and nurses in institutions for the insane" that had both classroom and field experience (Quiroga, 1995, p. 42). Eleanor Clark Slagle took this training course in 1911 and later began developing the profession of occupational therapy. In the next decade, several U.S. hospitals provided training courses on the use of occupations, but no official standards were developed until the U.S. Army established specific war emergency courses in 1918. The Surgeon General's office developed a 12- to 16-week training curriculum in September 1918 that included 264 hours of arts and crafts teaching, 64 hours of medical lectures, and 24 hours of hospital practice (Kearney, 2004).

The National Society for the Promotion of Occupational Therapy was formed in 1917, and in 1921 its name changed to the American Occupational Therapy Association (AOTA). One of the pressing needs at that time was to create national educational standards. The initial 1923 standards called for 9 months of classroom instruction, followed by at least 3 months of hospital training, called "hospital practice training" (comparable to fieldwork education). In 1927, a report of the Committee on Teaching Methods was given at the AOTA conference in Minneapolis (Privott, 1998). There were six schools of occupational therapy at that time whose training programs ranged from 9 months to 2 years, with hospital practice training ranging from the required 3 months to 9 months. The 1927 report addressed occupational therapists' transition from their schooling to the hospital setting:

> The step from school to hospital is a sudden one. The atmosphere
> and routine of the two are totally unlike. The student has been
> the center of interest in the school. The school with its faculty,
> curriculum, and equipment is organized to serve her. The hospital,
> on the other hand, is equipped and staffed to serve the patients.
> The patients have many needs of which occupational therapy is
> only one. The student from being considered, must now consider.
> The transition from school to hospital is attended with such real
> dangers to the student's powers of adjustment that both schools
> and hospitals have appreciated the value of giving the students
> some early contact with patients and some practical experience in
> dealing with the sick to prepare them for the hospital situation.
> (quoted in Privott, 1998, p. 294)

The Report of the Committee on Teaching Methods was read at the 11th annual meeting of the AOTA held in Minneapolis, Minnesota, in 1927 and stated the varied daily routines of hospital practice training. Students spent as much as 8 $^3/_4$ hours per day, or 48 hours per week, in the hospital. During the day, students rotated through the various wards but also attended lectures and had preparation time. The report concluded with the recommendation that hospital practice training be increased from 3 months to 6 months (cited in Privott, 1998, p. 431).

The earliest mention of the role of the supervisor in hospital practice training occurred at the 1927 AOTA conference in a statement made by a Miss Taylor, director of occupational therapy at the Robert B. Brigham Hospital in Boston, during the report of the Committee on Teaching Methods. She addressed the need for supervisors to be flexible in their training approach and suggested that students try to imitate their supervisors. Taylor also addressed the need for supervisors to be highly motivated and to commit themselves to this extra work:

> I feel that training as we are carrying it on is a service to the school and the progress of the profession, not a service to the hospital. Treatment as it is given our patients is of such great importance that the responsibility on the therapists is very great. It is not possible to shift that responsibility to young inexperienced students so they must always work under the guidance of the therapist. . . . I find the students very much like reflections in mirrors. We expect much of them and if we do not find them to be angels we forget that it is perhaps our reflection we are seeing, not the students. Every student presents an individual problem which must be solved as such. We can have a general outline of training, but I find that I must adapt my program to each separate group in order to do the most for that entire group. I believe that formal conferences are necessary as well as informal ones. When I chat with students in the shop during preparation time, I get and give much that is not possible in the more formal atmosphere of staff conference. The staff workers need to have their interest in training stimulated, not only at the beginning of the students' training, but every day the time the students are with us. Only this way is the extra burden of training of enough interest to them to make them give the most to it. (quoted in Privott, 1998, p. 439.)

In 1928, at the AOTA conference in Boston, a Dr. Hill from Worcester State Hospital gave a report titled "An Experiment in Clinical Affiliation for Occupational Therapy Students in a Mental Hospital," and in it the term *clinical affiliation* appeared for the first time. Hill described the purpose of fieldwork:

> Therapy being an art, this instruction is preliminary only to actual experience in hospitals treating such conditions. This actual contact, under experienced supervision, with patients being treated for the conditions previously studied develops the art of

occupational therapy. . . . The next logical step, of course, is the inclusion in the curriculum of the school of a period of practical training in a mental hospital where under experienced direction may be practiced the art of applying occupational therapy to the problem of the straightening out of a disordered personality. (quoted in Privott, 1998, p. 108)

Hill described the first cohort of eight occupational therapy students from the Boston School of Occupational Therapy, who spent 12 weeks at Worcester State Hospital for their clinical affiliation:

This program contemplates 579 hours of duty in twelve weeks—meaning five days of $8^3/_4$ hours each and a sixth of $4^1/_2$ hours. On time taken from the above schedule, each student also had a brief experience of assigned duty with patient groups for evening entertainments, including dances, moving pictures, athletics, etc. Each student also was excused from the regular schedule in order to attend for a time the regular hospital staff meetings and ward walks. There were conducted each Saturday morning a conference of the students with the superintendent of the hospital, wherein could be discussed any problems related to the work which the students wished to present. . . . [The students] came to us in the spirit of doubting adventure. At first they were counting the days, because for most of them it was a first experience with mental patients, with all the disturbance which that implies, and for most of them also the hardest work they had ever undertaken. It is one thing to be a visiting student and another to be a regular soldier in the line of duty. Later the students generally expressed the opinion that three months was not long enough to absorb the value which was in the experience. At the end of the three months they felt, as did we, that they were just ready to begin to assume responsibility and acquire that experience which comes in no other way. (quoted in Privott, 1998, p. 111)

Formal Standards for Clinical Supervision

In 1924, AOTA published the Minimum Standards for Courses of Training in Occupational Therapy. In 1931, however, AOTA requested that the American Medical Association take responsibility for the accreditation of occupational therapy educational programs. The resulting standards, titled "Essentials of an Acceptable School of Occupational Therapy," were adopted in 1935. This revised training curriculum, authored by the AMA, included 100 weeks of full-time training, including coursework in biological sciences, clinical conditions, social sciences, occupational therapy theory, electives, and instruction in major crafts. Clinical training was increased to a minimum of 36 weeks and specified requirements for the supervisor: "The hospital training of students must be supervised by a properly qualified, Registered occupational therapist, who is not only competent in her department, but has shown ability to handle students-in-training" (AOTA, quoted in Quiroga, 1995, p. 230).

The Committee on Student Affiliations was established as a subcommittee of the Council on Education by AOTA in 1941, thus changing the name from *hospital practice training* to *student affiliations*. It defined the purpose of affiliations as being to "promote closer correlation of the didactic preparation and clinical practice phases of occupational therapy education and to assure more uniform preparation for occupational therapy students" (AMA, 1943, p. 683). Until then, there was no standardization of clinical affiliation procedures. The 1943 Essentials made changes only to the content of the didactic portion of the training curriculum. In 1949 the Essentials were again revised to increase the length and vary the experiences of the clinical affiliations. Students were now required to spend 12 weeks in psychiatry, 8 weeks in a physical disabilities setting, 4–8 weeks in a tuberculosis setting, 4–8 weeks in pediatrics, and 4–8 weeks in general medicine and surgery.

AOTA issued publications that addressed supervision. The first was the *Manual for Supervisors of Student Affiliations,* which was intended for direct student supervisors (AOTA, 1948). This manual was revised in 1950, 1952, 1957, and 1962. The first page stated the sole requirement for becoming a student supervisor: "The therapist who serves as instructor must be a competent occupational therapist able to supervise students" (p. 1). The second publication was *A Director's Guide for a Clinical Training Program for Occupational Therapy Students,* prepared by the Sub-Committee on Clinical Training of the Committee on Education (AOTA, 1950). This guide was the first attempt within the profession to define the parameters of clinical supervision provided to students during fieldwork experiences. The minimum requirement for supervising students was to be registered or eligible for registration as an occupational therapist: "Registration is essential in keeping staff qualifications high and on a good professional level" (p. 2). This document underscored the importance of supervision during clinical training:

> The guidance of students during their training is one of the greatest responsibilities the director has to meet. The students are in the transition stage of becoming professional individuals. Adjustment, both professional and personal, must be guided by continual observations, consultation, and demonstration on the part of registered therapists." (p. 15)

The AOTA/AMA "Essentials of an Acceptable School of Occupational Therapy" were again revised in 1965, reducing the amount of clinical training from 36 weeks to 24 weeks, with 12 of those weeks to be in a psychosocial setting and 12 weeks to be in a physical dysfunction setting (cited in Kearney, 2004, p. 8). Published as the *Guide Book for an Accredited Curriculum in Occupational Therapy,* these new standards further defined the need for a bridge between the educational institution and the clinical site:

> 9. The Supervisor of Clinical Experience should be members of the faculty or extra-mural faculty of the college. They should be registered occupational therapists with a minimum of 2 years of clinical experience. In recognition of the concept of unification of academic and clinical instruction, the clinical supervisor should be identified as members of the instructional staff and be encouraged to participate in any way possible with the academic staff.
>
> Competency in clinical supervision should be recognized by an official faculty appointment with or without salary when appropriate within the policy of the institution. Competency should include knowledge of and ability to apply principles of learning in the clinical practice situation.
>
> In order that the clinical affiliation be educationally meaningful, it is imperative that the supervising therapist be skilled in patient evaluation, planning, integrating of patient treatment, departmental programming with allied professionals, be knowledgeable and skilled in teaching methods, guidance and supervision, and be familiar with the theoretical knowledge offered the student in his specific academic preparation. Active participation by the supervising therapist in the appropriate occupational therapy councils on basic professional education is essential. (AOTA, 1965, p. 13)

In the 1965 Eleanor Clarke Slagle lecture, titled "Learning as a Growth Process: A Conceptual Framework for Professional Education," Gail Fidler (1966) addressed the psychological processes inherent in the supervisory relationship of the practicum or clinical experience:

> Supervision is conceptualized as a dynamic teaching–helping relationship committed to the learning and growth of the student or supervisee. This learning experience has as its focus the exploration, analysis and synthesis of the ongoing functions of the learner to the extent that theoretical knowledge may emerge as a professional skill. It exists on the basis that learning must be a

conscious process in order for integration to be maximized and that self-awareness and understanding is the substructure of professional maturation and competency. Supervision in this sense becomes the primary modus operandi in fulfilling the educational aims of the clinical experience and such is the contract which binds supervisor and learner together. . . . This helping–teaching process needs to be an ongoing occurrence, regular scheduled and proceeding in a logical sequence related to the learner's individual capacities. Although what the student brings to the learning experience has an influence on the transaction, fulfillment of the supervisory contract will depend in great measure upon the attitudes and skill of the supervisor. The teaching–helping relationship, in the context for meeting professional expectations, has as one of its major goals increased self-awareness and understanding—perception and understanding of self not as a goal in itself but for the purpose of developing a coherent, definable set of constructs concerning the dynamics of interpersonal relationships and the assimilation of knowledge into basic attitudes and modes of functioning. The supervisor therefore must be free from biases to be able to approach situations realistically. He must possess an openness and receptivity to looking at feelings and their impact on behavior and have enough self-awareness and understanding to provide the assurance and objectivity so necessary to exploring and understanding ongoing function and catalyzing appropriate change. (Fidler, 1966, p. 7)

AOTA published *Student Affiliations* in 1966 to guide occupational therapists and occupational therapy students in the process of supervision during affiliations (AOTA, 1966b). It defined supervision as

a two-way communication process. The affiliate [student] can hasten his progress by a thoughtful use of supervision, particularly in the following areas:
a. Request guidance when necessary by asking pertinent questions.
b. Contribute to the overall functioning of the department by using personal resources and those available at the center.
c. Observe available experiences carefully and share ideas regarding change with the supervisor.
d. Observe proper channels of procedure regarding suggestions, criticism and grievances. (p. 6)

In 1971 AOTA published *Standards and Guidelines of an Occupational Therapy Affiliation Program*, which clearly delineated the requirements for supervision:

22. Supervision of Students

A. The student should be supervised in all aspects of his affiliation by adequate supervisory staff who should have full knowledge of the responsibility for all aspects of the program being carried out by a student under his aegis. "Actively supervised" means the supervisor should have full knowledge of the student's assigned caseload and responsibilities and how they are being handled.

B. The Clinical Education Supervisor should have a minimum of 2 years' clinical experience of which one should include supervision of students. The clinical education supervisor is the occupational therapist who is responsible for the total educational program in occupational therapy.

C. The registered occupational therapist who serves as a student supervisor must have a minimum of 1 year's practice in occupational therapy.

D. Supervision should be an ongoing daily and/or weekly process, an essential part of the program, and should be flexible in accordance with the patients, needs and abilities of the student. (AOTA, 1971, p. 316)

In 1975, AOTA published *Guidelines for Developing a Fieldwork Experience Program*, the first time that "fieldwork" was used to describe clinical training. This document also included a provision to allow for non–occupational therapy staff to supervise in settings with no occupational therapist on staff:

4. A registered occupational therapist with no less than 1 year of experience in direct service to patients/clients shall have responsibility for the student educational program and professional growth.

5. In those settings where no registered occupational therapist is on site, an appropriate professional certified by his profession and employed in the field setting, shall be the on-site administrative supervisor and shall assume responsibility for the students functioning within the setting. Such a professional shall not replace nor be in lieu of the registered occupational therapy supervisor as described above. This professional shall be familiar with the objectives of the fieldwork experience

and shall collaborate with the registered occupational therapy supervisor to ensure achievement of the educational objectives. "Appropriate professionals" may include teachers, social workers, public health nurses, ministers, probation officers, physical therapists, and the like. (p. 494)

In 1977, AOTA published the *Fieldwork Experience Manual for Academic Fieldwork Coordinators, Fieldwork Supervisors, and Students* as an interim document of the Commission on Education. This publication defined and described the supervision that should occur in occupational therapy fieldwork:

Supervision is an educational endeavor. The ultimate purpose of supervision is to direct the preparation of the student towards a given level of functioning as an occupational therapist. As such, supervision is both planned and modified with time. First, individualized goals and objectives are identified. Then the student is assisted to develop problem-solving skills through the gradual accumulation of experience and the quantitative additional responsibility for seeking out supervision when needed and for being self-directed. When the student has exhausted individual possibilities, supervision should encourage the exploration of other alternatives to expand the student's versatility and sophistication in the application of theoretical knowledge. Supervision has two related albeit separate aspects in relation to the accomplishment of learning goals and objectives . . . .

In fieldwork education, supervision is concerned with developing professional identity in the student which will facilitate the assumption of professional role functioning in occupational therapy. Supervision is thus conceptualized as (1) a dynamic teaching–learning relationship, (2) an educational process which serves as a bridge between previously learned knowledge and skill, and (3) a mechanism which insures an ongoing experiential learning environment. Within these concepts, the supervisor is a facilitator of learning who serves both as a reflective and evaluative mode to the student as progress is made toward self-responsibility relative to the professional role as an occupational therapist.

In summary, the supervisory relationship is a collaborative one in which both participants assume responsibility for (1) identifying the student's specific needs and goals, and (2) formulating a plan of growth which leads to the achievement of professional competence. The student and supervisor, working together, can develop a supervisory relationship in which both are comfortable relating problems and difficulties so that solutions can be mutually effected. The focus and boundaries of the relationship must be comparatively developed in order that both participants enjoy a productive experience. (pp. 13–14)

The *Essentials* were revised again in 1983 and introduced Level I fieldwork experiences in addition to Level II fieldwork experiences. Level I fieldwork was to be linked to didactic coursework so that students were exposed to the concepts they had been learning in the classroom (Kierney, 2004, p. 9). The *Essentials*, now called *Educational Programs: Essentials of an Accredited Educational Program for the Occupational Therapist* and *Educational Programs: Essentials of an Accredited Educational Program for the Occupational Therapy Assistant* (AOTA, 1983a, 1983b), again were revised in 1991; this draft was the last of the *Essentials* to be published by the Committee on Allied Health Education and Accreditation (CAHEA) and the AMA. The *Essentials* that were revised in 1995 only made mention of a new accrediting body, the Accreditation Council for Occupational Therapy Education (ACOTE), and did not mention any curricular changes, nor were there any changes were made to fieldwork education.

AOTA revised the *Fieldwork Experience Manual for Academic Fieldwork Coordinators, Fieldwork Supervisors, and Students* in 1984, expanding the section on supervision:

This expansion is in recognition of the growing appreciation of the impact that supervisory relationships have on the course of the fieldwork experience. Recent literature indicates that one of the most significant aspects of the fieldwork experience is the relationship between the student and the fieldwork educator. (p. iii)

Two more recent AOTA publications provide guided instruction to fieldwork educators on the process of clinical supervision for students during fieldwork: *Self-Paced Instruction for Clinical Education and Supervision* (SPICES; Crepeau & LaGarde, 1991) and *Meeting the Fieldwork Challenge* (AOTA, 2000), a self-study program. The former listed the four functions of the fieldwork educator role as follows:

1. *Administrative*—to enable the student to fulfill fieldwork objectives;
2. *Teaching*—to stimulate a student's desire to learn;
3. *Consultative*—to develop the student's confidence; and
4. *Evaluative*—to provide assessments to foster personal and professional development as well as meet academic requirement. (Ryan, 1991, p. 141)

Meeting the Fieldwork Challenge reflected the growing awareness of adult learning theories as fundamental in the fieldwork education process: "Fieldwork education relies on a different set of teaching strategies. . . . Fieldwork education should primarily provide pragmatic learning opportunities to transition skills from classroom to practice and to generalize practice competencies to a variety of related conditions" (AOTA, 2000, p. 4). This document stressed the importance of lifelong learning:

> The art of being a fieldwork educator is grounded in the desire to be a perpetual student. Fieldwork educators are always learning something new—from books, workshops, advanced education, and even from fieldwork students. To be effective, a fieldwork educator must highly value education and lifelong learning as a professional goal. (p. 9)

This chapter has reviewed the tremendous growth of our profession in meeting the educational needs of students since the early 1900s, when the profession of occupational therapy began. The evolution of fieldwork standards and requirements has had a rich history that has been responsive to both the changing needs identified within the profession and the changes in societal needs.

 Learning Activities

1. This chapter focused on the historical development of clinical supervision in the professions of medicine, social work, and occupational therapy. What similarities and differences did you notice among these professions in how they defined and developed clinical supervision?

2. Jantzen and Yerxa (1966; Yerxa, 1984) conducted workshops on the clinical experience. Some of the questions they asked workshop participants are still relevant today:

> One of the major things we consider in evaluating staff is the caliber of supervision given to the student from an educational point of view. The supervision you provide uses the tutorial method, so the intensity of the student–teacher relationship in the clinical experience is much closer than in other student–teacher relationships. It is very important, therefore, for us to know what kinds of people these are who supervise students and how they handle this relationship.

Now, how about your competence as a supervisor? Learning about people is a highly charged emotional experience." (Jantzen & Yerxa, 1966, pp. 53–54)

How do you handle this highly charged emotional experience?

3. "What are some of our responsibilities to the student during the fieldwork?" (Yerxa, 1984, p. 163).

4. "Reflect on your own past professional experiences for a moment. What experiences motivated you to pour more of yourself than you thought possible into study, thought, and hard work? Weren't there often moments when you contacted a person who represented a high level of professional competency, enthusiasm, and respect for truth?" (Yerxa, 1984, p. 169).

5. "If we open communications with students, we have to expect to run across some problems we cannot cope with. What do we do then?" (Yerxa, 1984, p. 172).

6. "We might ask ourselves, what can fieldwork educators do to make the fieldwork experience meaningful and educational for the student? What do we hope to accomplish? Why? How do we intend to accomplish it? What can we do to shoulder this heavy responsibility effectively?" (Yerxa, 1984, p. 162).

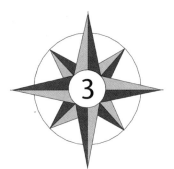

Theoretical Models of Supervision

*One can imitate an outstanding supervisor, but without theory or a
conceptual model, one does not really understand the process of supervision.*

(Hart, 1982, p. 27)

This chapter focuses on models of clinical supervision that have developed
over the past several decades. Some are influenced by adult learning theories,
some by psychological frames of reference, and still others by different philosophical orientations and approaches to supervision. Just as in the field of occupational therapy there are numerous frames of reference that guide treatment
interventions, different theoretical models of clinical supervision guide how
occupational therapists supervise. Theories, models, and frames of reference
help supervisors make sense of an overwhelming amount of information and
synthesize it into a framework that guides problem-solving and decision making. A *model* is, in essence, "a description of what something is and how it
works. A model of supervision is a theoretical description of what supervision
is and how the supervisee's learning and professional development occur"
(Haynes, Corey, & Moulton, 2003, p. 109).

Campbell (2000), in her book *Essentials of Clinical Supervision,* discussed
some popular approaches to supervision that are not grounded in theory. The
first is the "no-model model"; clinicians become supervisors simply by virtue of
being good clinicians. Being a good clinician, however, does not necessarily
imply that one is a good supervisor. Supervision is an intervention in its own
right, with a specific body of knowledge and theoretical perspectives.
Supervisors using the no-model model have had no formal training in how to
supervise students and frequently decide to supervise students the same way
their supervisors supervised them. This approach can lead to a management-by-
crisis approach, with the supervisor responding to students' cries for help when
they become overwhelmed. No real planning goes into this approach, and
learning is haphazard at best.

The "expert model" is a top-down approach to supervision that is tradi-
tionally used in the medical field (Campbell, 2006, p. 36). The supervisor is the
expert, and the student is a blank slate who is told what is right and what is
wrong. I often call this model the "mini-me model," because the idea is to have
the student imitate the supervisor. There is no collaboration in this model, and
students are expected to be passive learners in the process.

In the "one-size-fits-all model," all students are treated the same, and supervisors use the same techniques and learning activities and expect the same rate of progression (Campbell, 2006, p. 37). This model ignores both adult learning theories and the occupational therapy profession's accreditation standards, which call for a more individualized approach to student learning. Finally, in the "student-as-patient model," supervision is conducted more like a psychotherapy session than supervision, with the task of the supervisor to "fix" the student.

Campbell (2006) highlighted the outcomes of these popular approaches to supervision. But more useful models of clinical supervision have been written about and studied for decades. Bernard and Goodyear (2004) categorized models of supervision into three groups: (1) those grounded in psychotherapy theories, (2) those grounded in developmental theories, and (3) those grounded in social role theories. I would add a fourth category, which contains two models—the Schwartz occupational therapy fieldwork model of ego stage development and the situational leadership model.

Psychotherapy-Based Models of Supervision

Bernard and Goodyear (2004) described a number of models of supervision based on theories of psychotherapy. Although there are literally hundreds of psychotherapeutic methods and techniques, only a handful have resulted in clearly delineated models of supervision. This section briefly summarizes these models; interested readers can consult the references cited for more detailed information.

Psychodynamic Model

The influence of Freudian ego psychology extended from the practice of psychoanalysis and psychotherapy into supervision, particularly in the fields of social work, psychology, and psychiatry. Some consider Freud to have been the first psychotherapy supervisor (Bernard & Goodyear, 2004). According to Frawley-O'Dea and Sarnat (2000, quoted in Bernard & Goodyear, 2004),

> Freud was the first supervisor and thus represents the archetypal supervisor to whom we all maintain a transference of some kind. In his model of supervision, he combined a positivistic stance analogous to his model of treatment with a personal insistence on maintaining a position as the ultimate arbiter of truth, knowledge, and power. (p. 77)

The goal of supervision in the psychodynamic model is to help supervisees develop therapeutic competence and acquire clinical expertise in working with patients while working on their own personal growth. The supervisor creates a learning alliance with the supervisee to promote the development of therapeutic skills and self-awareness. Supervision feels more like personal psychotherapy than educationally oriented supervision; the intrapsychic processes of the supervisee are examined in the context of the relationship with the patient and with the supervisor in what is referred to as the *therapeutic triad*. As Cara and MacRae (2005) described it, "The therapist identifies with his or her patient and then elicits emotion in the supervisor that he or she experienced with the patient" (p. 658).

Person-Centered Model

The person-centered supervisory model evolved out of the work of pioneering humanistic psychologist Carl Rogers, who reportedly was the first person to report using transcribed interviews in supervision rather than just the supervisee's recollections (Bernard & Goodyear, 2004, p. 79). This model also has been referred to as *humanistic* or *facilitative supervision* (Cara & MacRae, 2005, p. 658). Person-centered supervision as Rogers described it is similar to the psychodynamic model in that supervisory sessions are similar to personal psychotherapy. Rogers believed that genuineness, warmth, and empathy are necessary not only for patients in therapy, but for supervisees as well:

> I think my major goal is to help the therapist grow in self-confidence and to grow in understanding of himself or herself, and to grow in understanding of the therapeutic process. And to that end, I find it very fruitful to explore any difficulties the therapist may feel that he or she is having working with the client. Supervision for me becomes a modified form of the therapeutic interview. (quoted in Bernard & Goodyear, 2004, p. 79)

Thus, through supervision, supervisees are given the opportunity to experience the same empathy and unconditional positive regard that characterize Rogerian therapy (Cara & MacRae, 2005, p. 658).

Cognitive–Behavioral Model

As the name implies, the cognitive–behavioral model of clinical supervision evolved out of the behavioral and cognitive–behavioral schools of psychotherapy. The emphasis in clinical supervision is on helping the supervisee gain skills such as goal setting in behavioral terms through role modeling and coaching (Cara & MacRae, 2005, p. 659). Boyd (1978, quoted in Bernard & Goodyear, 2004) identified propositions central to cognitive–behavioral supervision:

1. Proficient therapist performance is more a function of learned skills than a "personality fit." The purpose of supervision is to teach appropriate therapist behaviors and extinguish inappropriate behavior.

2. The therapist's professional role consists of identifiable tasks, each one requiring specific skills. Training and supervision should assist the trainee in developing these skills, applying and refining them.

3. Therapy skills are behaviorally definable and are responsive to learning theory, just as there are other behaviors.

4. Supervision should employ the principles of learning theory within its procedures. (p. 80)

Just as in cognitive–behavioral therapy where the therapist assigns goals to clients, in cognitive–behavioral supervision the supervisor assigns learning tasks to the supervisee. This form of supervision also relies heavily on the Socratic method of questioning to increase learning.

Systemic Model

The systemic model of clinical supervision is based on family systems theory and is most relevant to therapists providing family therapy. According to this model, family dynamics are replicated in the supervisory session (Bernard & Goodyear, 2004). The supervisor takes a very active role in collaborating with the supervisee. Occupational therapists working with families or individuals on family-of-origin issues should use supervision to explore and resolve their own family-of-origin issues:

> The activation of family-of-origin dynamics is a supervision issue because they affect the degree of objectivity and emotional reactivity that counselors have with their clients and hence their therapeutic capabilities. . . . Therefore, supervision should provide trainees with opportunities to attain higher levels of differentiation and emotional maturity. (2001, Montgomery, Hendricks, & Bradley, 2001, quoted in Bernard & Goodyear, 2004, p. 82)

Constructivist Models

Constructivist supervision is an umbrella term for several psychotherapy-based models that focus on the meaning one makes out of life experiences. In these models, supervision takes on a more consultative role (Bernard & Goodyear, 2004). There are two distinct models of supervision in this category—narrative approaches to supervision and solution-focused supervision—each corresponding to the type of psychotherapy of the same name.

As the name implies, the narrative approach to therapy uses a storytelling technique to help clients organize their life events and experiences. Clients come to therapy to tell their story, and it is the therapist's job to listen and help them tell that story. Novice occupational therapists are in the process of developing their own professional life story, and supervision is a process of revising the stories that trainees (1) tell about their clients (i.e., a *metastory*), (2) tell about themselves, and (3) tell about their other therapists. The role of the supervisor, then, is to serve as an editor or catalyst to help trainees define who they are as therapists and what they do in that role. (Bernard & Goodyear, 2004, p. 84)

In solution-focused therapy, the emphasis is not on what is wrong with clients but rather on helping them get what they want out of life. There is a primary assumption that clients know what is best for themselves and that there is more than one solution to problems, and the focus is on what can change and what is possible (Bernard & Goodyear, 2004). This form of therapy uses what is referred to as the "miracle question": "Imagine that a miracle has occurred: The problems for which you are seeking treatment magically disappear. What, *specifically*, will you notice that will tell you this has occurred?" (p. 84). Similarly, in supervision, the supervisor helps the supervisee discover his or her own strengths and resources. There is an emphasis on working with the supervisee's successes rather than pointing out shortcomings. The supervisor might use the following questions in supervision: "Tell me, what have you done better this week in working with your clients?" or "What was the best intervention you provided to one of your clients since we last met?" If the supervisee resists and wants to focus on his or her shortcomings, the supervisor might use a variation of the miracle question, such as "Imagine you have completed your Level II fieldwork successfully—what changes might you have made in how you work with clients in this setting?"

Developmental Models of Supervision

Developmental models of clinical supervision share the focus of looking at supervisees' professional development as they progress through clearly defined stages.

Integrated Development Model

Psychologist and professor Cal D. Stoltenberg and his colleagues described the integrated development model, which has gone through several revisions (Bernard & Goodyear, 2004). It is the best known and most widely used of all the developmental models. Stoltenberg and associates described eight domains of professional functioning or competency that supervisees must develop: (1) intervention skills, (2) assessment techniques, (3) interpersonal assessment, (4) client conceptualization, (5) individual differences, (6) theoretical orientation, (7) treatment plans and goals, and (8) professional ethics. According to this model, professional development moves through four stages in each domain, and each stage involves dimensions of professional growth: (1) self–other awareness, (2) motivation, and (3) autonomy. In Level 1, supervisees have limited training or limited experience. Their motivation is high, but so is their anxiety. They want to gain the skills necessary for effective practice, and they want to know the "best" approach. In terms of autonomy, they are dependent on their supervisor, require structure and positive feedback, and cannot tolerate confrontation. Their self–other awareness is limited: They are focused on themselves, but they lack self-awareness and are anxious about being evaluated.

Level 2 supervisees are in transition from being dependent to imitating their supervisors. Their motivation fluctuates, and they alternate between being very confident and appearing confused. Supervisees at Level 2 are more autonomous, but they still vacillate between dependence and independence. Their awareness focuses more on the other—namely, their clients. However, they need assistance from their supervisors in maintaining a healthy balance. Level 2 supervisees can be challenging for supervisors because of their inconsistencies, and a flexible approach is recommended.

Level 3 supervisees are developing a clearer sense of themselves as occupational therapists and understand better their role in the therapeutic process. Their motivation is more consistent; although they have some doubts, they are not overwhelmed by these doubts. Level 3 supervisees have developed more autonomy and are able to trust their own professional judgment. They can be more collegial in supervisory sessions with their supervisors because their anxieties have diminished. Their self–other awareness has increased, and they are able to focus on their clients and to monitor their own personal reactions to their clients.

The last stage is called Level 3i, or *integrated;* the supervisee has achieved most of the competencies necessary for entry-level practice. They are well aware of their strengths and weaknesses (Bernard & Goodyear, 2004).

Ronnestad and Skovholt Model

Unlike other theoretical models, the one developed by psychologist Michael Helge Ronnestad and educational psychologist Thomas M. Skovholt (2005) was based on interviews with 100 counselors and therapists whose experience varied from still being in graduate school to being 40 years out of training. This model supports the notion of lifelong learning in that the phases it identifies extend throughout a professional career. On the basis of these interviews, they identified six phases of therapist development.

Phase 1 is the lay helper phase and usually occurs before trainees enter a professional training program. They may do volunteer service work or observe an occupational therapist with the intention of entering an occupational therapy educational program. Trainees in this phase typically have had some experience with helping others, such as friends or family members. Because they have no formal training or supervision, they may have difficulty establishing and maintaining interpersonal boundaries with clients; they tend to overidentify with those they help, expressing sympathy instead of empathy.

In Phase 2, the beginning student phase, supervisees are excited at the prospect of beginning to learn the theory and practice of their chosen profession. They begin to visit clinical sites, as in Level I fieldwork experiences. They are dependent on the supervisor for direction and support and may appear anxious and confused at times. Some have difficulty receiving negative feedback or constructive criticism, which may undermine their fragile self-confidence. However, they are eager to learn, often express a desire to become just like their supervisors, and seek to discover the one best way to work with clients.

Students in Phase 3, the advanced student phase, have completed the bulk of the didactic portion of their professional training and are beginning their internships in Level II fieldwork. Initially, they often experience a self-induced pressure to perform correctly at all times, resulting in an anxious appearance and formal, almost rehearsed conversation. They are aware that they have acquired a beginning level of knowledge but feel vulnerable because they have not yet integrated that knowledge. Supervision that is supportive and that confirms what students already know works best in this phase. Supervisors need to be proficient at bolstering confidence by asking questions to which the student will be able to respond. One way to help students in this phase feel more confident is to assign them tasks such as orienting new students or letting beginning-level students observe them. They often report that such tasks made them aware that they knew more than they thought they knew.

Phase 4, the novice professional phase, is the beginning of entry-level practice for most health care professionals. They have successfully completed the didactic and clinical portions of their training programs, but they often feel that they have just scratched the surface of the professional body of knowledge. Students are anxious at this stage to begin working, but they should be strongly encouraged to obtain clinical supervision to manage the steep learning curve ahead of them. During the first few years of practice, supervisees begin to integrate their personalities into their interventions with clients, discovering their own best way to work with clients. They often do not stay at their first job very long; they are in the process of discovering what practice environment they prefer to work in and with whom.

In Phase 5, the experienced professional phase, occupational therapists have begun to relax after the first few years of practice and to truly come into their own, discovering ways they can fully integrate their personalities, values, and interests into their professional lives. They have become comfortable with establishing and maintaining therapeutic relationships with clients, and they are able to engage clients actively in the treatment process and lead them to change. Supervisees at this level begin to understand that they can learn a great deal from their clients. They also begin to supervise students, which for some can fulfill a sense of professional commitment, a kind of giving back to the profession. It is extremely important that they continue to obtain some supervision, because providing supervision is unfamiliar territory for most. Unless they have had formal training in clinical supervision, practitioners tend to imitate their earlier experiences of supervision, either emulating great supervisors or repeating the mistakes of less-than-optimal supervisors.

Practitioners in Phase 6, the senior professional phase, typically have more than 20 years' experience in their profession. They have developed very individualized styles of working with their clients, feel secure in the way they work, and appear very modest about their impact on their clients' lives. Depending on their career trajectory, some may be burned out, whereas others have become wise masters. They may or may not have continued their commitment to lifelong learning and may welcome or reject new developments in the field. Other personal forces in their lives may lead them to make career changes, return to school, tend to family issues, or contemplate retirement. Supervision can be critical at this point, but many practitioners in this phase no longer are engaged in their own supervision because they are too busy supervising others. Supervision can help seasoned occupational therapists make decisions about career moves, rediscover their passions, and avoid burnout (Bernard & Goodyear, 2004).

In addition to these six phases, Ronnestad and Skovholt (2003) identified 14 themes in therapist development:

1. Professional development involves an increasing higher-order integration of the professional self and the personal self.
2. The focus shifts dramatically over time, from internal to external to internal.
3. Continuous reflection is a pre-requisite for optimal learning and professional development at all levels of experience.
4. An intense commitment to learn propels the developmental process.
5. The cognitive map changes: Beginning practitioners rely on external expertise, and seasoned practitioners rely on internal expertise.
6. Professional development is a long, slow, continuous process that can also be erratic.
7. Professional development is a lifelong process.
8. Many beginning practitioners experience much anxiety in their professional work. Over time, anxiety is mastered by most.
9. Clients serve as the major source of influence and serve as primary teachers.
10. Personal life influences professional functioning and development throughout the professional life span.
11. Interpersonal sources of influence propel professional development more than "impersonal" sources of influence.

12. New members of the field view professional elders and graduate training with strong affective reactions.
13. Extensive experience with suffering contributes to heightened recognition, acceptance, and appreciation of human variability. The authors were referring to the developmental process therapists go through to reach a state of wisdom and integrity. Novice supervisees often express how "bad" they feel working with people who are suffering; the authors label this as sympathy. Over time, the practitioner learns how to listen to the suffering with empathy rather than sympathy— how to distance him- or herself from the pain and suffering to be truly helpful to the client. The reader is referred to readings on compassion fatigue for more explanation.
14. For the practitioner there is realignment from Self as Hero to Client as Hero (Bernard & Goodyear, 2004).

Bernard and Goodyear (2004, p. 90) stated that these themes add to the "cognitive map" of clinical supervision and support the necessity of offering formal courses.

Loganbill, Hardy, and Delworth Model

The model developed by psychologists Carol Loganbill, Emily Hardy, and Ursula Delworth (1982) is familiar to occupational therapists and occupational therapy assistants because it has been described in many occupational therapy textbooks (e.g., AOTA, 1991; Cara & MacRae, 2005; Frum & Opacich, 1987). These authors were among the first to propose a model of clinical supervision and professional development. Their model consists of three stages that describe how supervisees view the world, themselves, and their supervisors. It is not a linear model but rather a circular, dynamic one, suggesting that supervisees will move through the cycle repeatedly throughout their careers.

Stage 1 is stagnation. Supervisees may report feeling stuck or unsure of how to proceed. Beginning students at this level are more likely to be unaware of any difficulties and, when asked to identify issues in supervision sessions, will respond that "everything's fine." Thinking in this stage is characterized by dichotomous black-or-white thinking. They may see only one way to respond to a situation and cannot generate alternatives. Students may demonstrate "a false sense of security. The environment seems deceptively stable and safe" (Frum & Opacich, 1987, p. 3). They may alternate between appearing overconfident about their knowledge and abilities and claiming to have been inadequately prepared for fieldwork. Their self-concept may be low, and they may be dependent on the supervisor as the primary source of learning. Their attitude toward the supervisor at this stage is likely to be "one of idealizing him or her as an omniscient and omnipotent figure or being indifferent to the supervisor and considering him or her to be irrelevant" (Cara & MacRae, 2005, p. 666).

The primary task for the supervisor of students at this stage is to reassure them that they know more than they think they know. Supervisors need to tolerate fluctuating performance levels and not personalize any inappropriate behavior students display toward the supervisor. Supervisors need to explain situations in detail and to help students generate alternatives in problem-solving. Even when students appear overconfident, supervisors should not give them too much autonomy or independence, or they may become overwhelmed and frustrated.

Supervisees may enter Stage 2, confusion, either gradually or abruptly. This stage is characterized by confusion and instability: "The student, in attempting to find a balance, moves randomly, trying various options in order to find the right, or perfect answer" (Frum & Opacich, 1987, p. 4). Students at this level may appear confident at times and feel like a failure at other times. They are unaware of how others assess their level of competence.

The idealization of the supervisor that characterizes Stage 1 is replaced by the realization that the supervisor does not have all the answers. This realization may cause the supervisee to display anger, disappointment, or resentment toward the supervisor, whom they feel is supposed to have all the answers. It is particularly important during this stage for supervisors to recognize the developmental tasks at hand and not to personalize the student's reactions to him or her. It also is helpful if the supervisor can help the student recognize and verbalize that this period and the corresponding emotions are an expected stage in the developmental process of becoming an occupational therapist.

The transition to Stage 3, integration, can be brief and abrupt or a more gradual process. Frum and Opacich (1987) described this stage as "the calm after the storm" (p. 4). The student is better able to understand the complexity of situations and to independently generate alternative solutions to problems. Supervisees are better able to use supervisory sessions and come prepared, having taken responsibility for their own learning. Their attitudes toward the supervisor also have changed to a more realistic view; just as supervisees now recognize their own strengths and weaknesses, they recognize those of the supervisor. The relationship changes to a more collegial one, as the mutual recognition of a peer relationship develops between the two. The supervisor can now introduce other issues into the supervisory sessions, such as ethics, advanced practice, and professional development. The supervisor can begin to challenge the student with more independence and autonomy while continuing to provide feedback on performance.

In addition to three stages of development in this model, Loganbill and colleagues (1982) identified eight basic supervisory issues that student trainees must address: (1) competence, (2) emotional awareness, (3) purpose and direction, (4) autonomy, (5) respect for individual differences, (6) professional ethics,

(7) motivation, and (8) identity. These are not sequential, as are the three stages, but rather are revisited within each stage.

One last component of the Loganbill and colleagues (1982) model comprises five supervisory interventions to help supervisees move through the developmental stages: (1) facilitative, (2) confrontive, (3) conceptual, (4) prescriptive, and (5) catalytic. The reader is referred to Loganbill and colleagues for detailed descriptions of these interventions.

Social Role Models of Supervision

Social role models of clinical supervision are characterized by their emphasis on the various professional roles in performing supervision. These models developed out of the recognition that supervision is a distinct intervention and that it is a higher-order role than teaching, counseling, or therapy: "Supervision is a separate skill similar to teaching—but different; similar to counseling—but different; and similar to consulting—but different" (Douce, 1989, quoted in Bernard & Goodyear, 2004, p. 94).

Discrimination Model

Bernard created the discrimination model of clinical supervision in 1979, when she was still a doctoral student and needed a model to teach a supervision course to graduate students (Bernard & Goodyear, 2004). This model describes the three roles that a supervisor chooses when trying to reach a goal in supervision: (1) teacher, (2) consultant, and (3) counselor. The discrimination model works with any theoretical orientation; it is independent of any psychological theory or model. Supervisors function in the teacher role when they ask content-oriented questions; give assignments; and review techniques, modalities, and theories. In the consultant role, the supervisor may review alternative models, suggest resources to explore, and encourage the supervisee to "think outside the box." The counselor role focuses more on the intrapersonal and interpersonal processes; the supervisor may ask the supervisee reflective questions to encourage him or her to identify feelings or recognize personal issues that may be interfering with therapy.

In addition, Bernard described three foci of supervision that are emphasized in supervision: (1) intervention skills, (2) conceptualization skills, and (3) personalization skills. In other words, the roles are the *how* of supervision, and the foci are the *what* of supervision. Intervention skills involve the treatments, modalities, and techniques the supervisee uses in therapy sessions with clients. Conceptualization skills focus on how the supervisee views the client's case, including the themes or processes he or she identifies. Personalization skills are what has been called the *therapeutic use of self*—in other words, how supervisees use themselves within therapy sessions with clients (Bernard & Goodyear, 2004).

Hawkins and Shohet Model

Organizational learning and culture researcher Peter Hawkins and psychotherapist Robin Shohet (2000) created a model of clinical supervision that has been called the *double matrix* or *seven-eyed model* of supervision, referring to the multiple phenomena present or levels operating in supervision. The authors identified the four elements in any supervision session: (1) the supervisee, (2) the supervisor, (3) the client, and (4) the work context. They theorized that there are two interlocking systems, or matrixes—the therapy system and the supervisory system. Both systems exist "within a wider context which impinges upon and colors the processes within it" (Hawkins & Shohet, 2000, p. 71). The processes, or modes of focus, that are explored in supervision are as follows:

- *Mode 1:* the content of the occupational therapy session
- *Mode 2:* the strategies and interventions provided
- *Mode 3:* the therapy relationship between the supervisee and the client
- *Mode 4:* the supervisee's internal process
- *Mode 5:* the supervisory relationship
- *Mode 6:* the supervisor's own process (Mode 6a is the supervisor–client relationship, an indirect relationship because usually the two have no direct contact. Hawkins and Shohet [2000] referred to this as a "fantasy relationship.")
- *Mode 7:* the wider context of the professional community in which the supervisor and supervisee practice.

The Hawkins and Shohet (2000) model also includes six factors that influence the choice of focus in supervision:

1. The nature and work of the therapist;
2. The style of the therapist's work;
3. The personality and learning style of the therapist;
4. The degree of openness and trust that has been established in the supervision relationship;
5. The amount of personal exploration the therapist has done for themselves (e.g., have they been in therapy?);
6. The cultural background of the therapist. (p. 87).

Holloway Systems Model

Psychologist and researcher Elizabeth Holloway's (1995) systems model is one of the newest. It is similar to Bernard and Goodyear's (2004) discrimination model in that it takes into account both the *what* and the *how* of supervision. The *what* of supervision is the tasks, and the *how* of supervision is the functions. Psychologist and professor Elizabeth Holloway listed the tasks of supervision as monitoring or evaluating, instructing or advising, modeling, consulting, and supporting or sharing. The functions of supervision are counseling skill, case conceptualization, professional role, emotional awareness, and self-evaluation (cited in Bernard & Goodyear, 2004, p. 99). This model combines the tasks and functions into a 5 x 5 matrix, with a total of 25 different combinations.

Other Models of Supervision

Schwartz Ego Stage Model

Clinical researcher Kathleen Barker Schwartz's (1984) ego stage model first appeared in the occupational therapy literature in 1984 and has been referenced in other texts since then (Cara & MacRae, 2005; Privott, 1998). It is the only clinical supervision model for fieldwork that was first described in the occupational therapy literature. The model is based on developmental theory, specifically that of Loevinger (1977). Loevinger conceptualized nine stages of ego state development across the life span, and Schwartz felt that three—Levels 3, 3/4, and 4—were most relative to fieldwork education.

Students at Level 3, the conscientious stage, view their supervisors as experts; they conform to external rules and feel guilty when they break the rules. A sense of belonging is important to them, and their interpersonal style is often superficial. Teaching should focus on presenting information in a factual manner and highlighting that there can be more than one solution. Supervision needs to provide clear structure, with defined expectations and assignments. Students are compliant at this stage; they want to please the supervisor and be accepted.

Level 3/4, the explorer stage, is characterized by increased awareness of self and others as the student matures in his or her helping role. The student is able to see multiple possibilities and alternatives but still expresses personal beliefs in a rigid way. Students may question their supervisors if the information presented does not fit with their conceptualizations. Teaching should reflect that students are capable of generating their own system of problem solving and should encourage students to accept opposing viewpoints. Supervision should use negotiation, allowing the student some input. Rules should be made clear, but students should realize that they will sometimes need to break the rules and that there may be consequences for breaking the rules. Supervisors should provide reassurance if students get upset when things do not go according to plan.

Students at Level 4, the achiever stage, demonstrate high levels of conceptual skill and can accept multiple opposing viewpoints. They are able to set long-term goals for themselves and can self-evaluate performance. Students are much more skilled at problem solving and can discover their own solutions when faced with a conflict. Supervisors can challenge students at this stage by asking them to explain the rationale behind their ideas and to defend or discuss the implications of their decisions. Collaboration between supervisor and supervisee is very effective at this stage, although students may argue over certain expectations. Support will be necessary when students experience failure, because they are hypercritical of themselves and easily prone to guilt at this stage.

Situational Leadership Model

The situational leadership model is based on the work of organizational scientist Paul Hersey, who originally developed the model in the 1960s and later developed it in collaboration with colleagues (Hersey, Blanchard, & Johnson, 1996). This model is not presented in most textbooks on clinical supervision, but I include it here because at least two applications of this model have been reported in the clinical education literature—one in nursing (Keenan, Hoover, & Hoover, 1988) and the other in athletic training (Meyer, 2000). This leadership model focuses on how leaders motivate, facilitate, and encourage people to reach their highest level of performance. What is unique about the model is that it addresses the impact of both the task and the person's motivation on performance. Hersey and colleagues described four leadership styles that have been adapted into supervisory styles or functions: (1) telling (or directing), (2) selling (or coaching), (3) participating (or supporting), and (4) delegating. In situational leadership, the supervisor adapts his or her behavior to match the situation or task at hand with the motivation or readiness of the supervisee.

Meyer (2000) described student behavior variables that determine which of the situational leadership styles is used:

- Level of emotional maturity,
- Level of cognitive ability,
- Level of motivation,
- Level of experience and confidence, and
- Level of efficacy in transferring knowledge to application.

The task of the supervisor is to assess the student's level of readiness via observation or written assessment and then use the approach that will provide the most appropriate level of challenge and promote the most growth for the student. The styles of telling and selling are recommended for students at the beginning of their student fieldwork experiences, whereas the participating and delegating styles may be more appropriate for advanced students. This model echoes what occupational therapy practitioners call the *just-right challenge*. Supervisors want the assignments they give their students to be hard or complex enough to be a bit of a reach, but not so easy that students feel that the work is beneath them or so difficult that they become frustrated and give up.

The following list examines the four styles in terms of student behaviors and fieldwork educator responses:

1. *Telling (or directing):* Students present with a low level of readiness; they feel insecure about their abilities or knowledge base. Fieldwork educators respond by providing clear, explicit instructions to students, minimizing the amount of decision making they have to do. Supervisors provide close supervision to students.

2. *Selling (or coaching):* Students demonstrate a moderate level of readiness; they still doubt their abilities, but they are willing to try to perform the assigned task. Supervisors explain the rationale behind treatment decisions, provide students with opportunities to ask questions, and provide a moderate level of guidance and supervision.

3. *Participating (or supporting):* Students demonstrate a moderate level of readiness; they feel able to perform the assigned task but still feel insecure in their abilities. Supervisors respond by sharing ideas, encouraging students to collaborate in the decision-making process, and providing moderate to low levels of supervision and guidance.

4. *Delegating:* Students' level of readiness is high; as they feel confident in their abilities. The fieldwork educator gives students more responsibility for decision making and carrying out treatment independently. They give students little guidance but adequate supervision.

This model is developmental in that it is individualized to each student and changes with the student's growth. It is appropriate for fieldwork supervision, because educators must demonstrate and model leadership for supervisees to help them adopt similar behaviors: "Situational leaders carry a substantial responsibility to lead and give power away as they encourage their followers in attaining their greatest potential" (Meyer, 2000, p. S264).

This chapter has provided readers with a review of the major theories and models of clinical supervision that have been developed across disciplines. It hopefully serves to underscore my contention that supervision is an intervention in its own right, grounded in a theory and knowledge base. Readers are encouraged to further their learning by reading more on those models that seem particularly relevant.

Learning Activities

1. Reflect on your own experiences of being supervised when you were a student. What aspects of the supervision were the most helpful to you? Which were the least helpful? What actions or assignments by your supervisor best facilitated learning? What would you have liked from your supervisor that you didn't get? What models or theories described in this chapter did your supervisor use? What can you learn from this reflection in designing your own model of supervision?

2. As you read through the descriptions of the various models presented in this chapter, which of them resonated with you? How might you use these models in your setting? Do some research and additional reading on those models to better understand them.

3. If you were starting all over as a student in the setting you are now working in, which model of supervision would you prefer your supervisor to use, and why?

4. How do you believe people learn best? How do you believe people can change and grow toward their highest potential? These beliefs about learning and personal growth will influence the model of clinical supervision you choose.

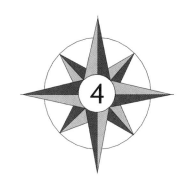

Effective Clinical Supervision

Good teachers, like good midwives, empower. Good teachers find ways to activate students, for they know that learning requires active engagement between the subject and "object matter." Learning requires discovery and invention. Good teachers know when to hang back and be silent, when to watch and wonder at what is taking place all around them. They can push and pull when necessary—just like midwives—but they know that they are not always called upon to perform. Sometimes the performance is and must be elsewhere, sometimes the teacher can feel privileged just to be present at the drama happening nearby.

(Ayers, 1986, p. 50)

This chapter reviews research in the fields of medicine, counseling, physical therapy, and occupational therapy on the qualities and characteristics of effective and ineffective clinical supervision. Learning about what students, academic faculty members, and clinical educators have said about ineffective and ineffective learning practices is one way clinical supervisors can improve their skills.

Clinical Supervision in Medicine

Clinical education is an essential component of medical students and residents' professional education, and yet one researcher has compared the variable quality of clinical education to minestrone soup—"lots of little bits, all chopped up, floating in a sea of indeterminate nutritional value" (Jolly, 1999, p. 86). In a study conducted in The Netherlands (van der Hem-Stokroos, Daelmans, van der Vleuten, Haarman, & Scherpbier, 2003), focus groups were conducted with medical students to determine the efficacy of their learning experiences. All of the students rated observation by physicians, particularly during patient encounters, as the most valuable learning experience. These students identified feedback provided as a key learning factor, adding that feedback needed to be provided in a positive manner (e.g., not being reprimanded in front of others), that the observer should have an openness toward asking questions, and that sensitive matters and negative feedback should be offered in private settings. Most students did not feel that they received adequate feedback. The article made several key recommendations, including active involvement of students in the learning process, increased direct observation, training for medical teaching staff on teaching methods, positive learning environments, and time for self-study.

Kilminster and Jolly (2000) reviewed the literature on the outcomes of effective clinical supervision across health professions. They found that supervision is the least investigated area of clinical education and that little theory or empirical evidence is available. In an article examining psychiatric residents' views on the psychotherapy supervision they received (Shanfield, Hetherly, & Matthews, 2001), the residents rated an accepting attitude and guidance in highly charged clinical dilemmas as the most valued characteristics of supervisors. Female residents were more critical of their supervisors than male residents, a finding that warrants further inquiry.

Hesketh and colleagues (2001) developed a curricular framework for facilitating the development of excellence in medical clinical education, recommending that medical educators take at least one course in teaching methods. The authors stated that recent developments in education, including a move away from the apprenticeship model to more experiential, problem-based learning model and increased systematic planning of the learning experience, led to this recommendation. Their curricular framework is based on a three-circle model in which the performance of tasks is framed by the approach to the tasks, with both of these relating to the professionalism and self-development of the medical teacher.

Clinical Supervision in Counseling

The mental health counseling professions—psychology, marriage and family counseling, and counseling—have conducted numerous studies on effective clinical supervision. They have produced some interesting results, but there have been methodological problems, including the inability to differentiate supervisee *satisfaction* from supervisee *effectiveness*. As Bernard and Goodyear (2004) observed, "To ask trainees about whether they were satisfied with supervision or their supervisor gives minimal information about the 'nutritional' value of their experience" (p. 10). Some studies have pointed out that qualities of the ideal supervisor are similar to qualities of the ideal therapist, including empathy, understanding, unconditional positive regard, genuineness, warmth, self-disclosure, flexibility, concern, attention, investment, curiosity, and being open (Hawkins & Shohet, 2000, p. 42). Psychologist Maria Gilbert and integrative psychotherapist Ken Evans (2001) identified a broader list of qualities, including flexibility, ability to view situations from multiple perspectives, multicultural competence, ability to contain one's own anxiety and that of the supervisee, openness to learning from new situations and from supervisees, ability to handle power appropriately, humor, humility, and patience.

Clinical psychologist and researcher Jen L. Lowry (2001, quoted in Haynes, Corey, & Moulton, 2003, pp. 64–65) studied psychologists and came up with lists of both effective and ineffective supervisory characteristics. The positive qualities included competency as a clinician, creation of an accepting supervisory climate, a desire to provide supervision, grading of supervision according to the supervisee's level of development, provision of constructive feedback, flexibility, availability to supervisees, and good relational skills. Negative characteristics include a judgmental attitude, a critical attitude toward the supervisee, rigidity, lack of commitment to supervision, poor clinical skills, unethical behavior or attitudes, poor boundaries, and self-absorption.

Campbell (2000) cited several studies reporting that supervisors should be confident but not dictatorial, should be respected by their colleagues, and should advocate for their supervisees. She quoted Virginia Satir, pioneering family therapist, as saying that "the better the supervisor's self-esteem, communication ability, personal congruence, and role flexibility, the more likely that the supervisory relationship will foster exploration, learning, and development" (quoted in Campbell, 2000, p. 5). The supervisor's ability to provide a supportive, facilitative environment is critical to the effectiveness of supervision, regardless of the supervisor's theoretical orientation. Campbell concluded with the observation that effective clinical supervisors focus on the student rather than on themselves.

Falender and Shafranske (2004) summarized an extensive body of research studies on high-quality supervision and formulated three categories of characteristics:

1. *Establishing a supportive relationship*—showing empathy; understanding the supervisee's struggles; cultivating a sense of teamwork between supervisor and supervisee; validating the supervisee; being approachable and flexible; being genuine; appearing interested in the supervisee; having a sense of humor; encouraging supervisee self-disclosure; providing regular and constructive feedback; being clear about expectations; and emphasizing personal growth, respect, inner harmony, and wisdom.
2. *Forming a working alliance*—agreeing on goals, collaborating, and encouraging trust and respect.
3. *Engaging in developmental supervision*—being sensitive to the developmental stages of the supervisee and making graded changes in supervision based on demonstrated growth in the supervisee.

Magnuson, Wilcoxon, and Norem (2000) discussed what they described as "lousy" supervision, identifying six categories of ineffective supervisory behaviors:

1. Focusing on small details and missing the big picture
2. Being developmentally inappropriate for the supervisee and providing static, unchanging supervision throughout the clinical experience

3. Being intolerant of differences and expecting the supervisee to imitate the supervisor
4. Providing poor role modeling of professional attributes, including violating boundaries with supervisees and judging them harshly
5. Neglecting to acquire training in supervision or teaching
6. Experiencing apathy and/or burnout or a lack of commitment to supervision.

Ellis (2001) also looked at harmful supervision, differentiating it from ineffective supervision in that the former causes trauma to the supervisee. Harmful supervision involves providing negligent supervision; engaging in malicious actions; violating professional ethics; engaging in sexual relationships with or sexually harassing supervisees; expressing demeaning or overcritical attitudes; publicly humiliating supervisees; and making derogatory remarks to supervisees of a sexist, racist, or ageist nature.

Nelson and Friedlander (2001) highlighted the power differential in the supervisory relationship and the vulnerability of the supervisee. In addition, they noted, supervisees often work long hours, experience anxiety about their performance, and are not always emotionally prepared to deal with the work of counseling. They concluded that supervisors need to be aware of the power issues in the relationship and to exercise great clinical skill in managing them. In addition, they recommended training for supervisors to enable them to develop alternate ways of handling supervisees' challenging behaviors.

Clinical Supervision in Physical Therapy

Strohschein, Hagler, and May (2002) underscored the importance of quality in clinical education to prepare future generations of physical therapists to commit to lifelong learning. Formal training of clinical educators, rather than trail-and-error learning, is essential, they observed. In addition, they noted that "expertise in clinical practice does not imply expertise in clinical education" (p. 162).

Physical therapist Michael J. Emery's landmark 1984 study identified 43 behaviors of clinical instructors that clustered into four categories: (1) communication, (2) interpersonal relationships, (3) professional skills, and (4) teaching behaviors (see Figure 4.1). The 102 physical therapy students they surveyed ranked communication as the most important attribute, followed by interpersonal skills, teaching skills, and professional skills.

Building on Emery's (1984) work, Cross (1995) examined the attributes of the ideal physical therapy clinical educator, comparing student attitudes with those of clinical educators and academic faculty. The three groups were asked to rank order the top six characteristics from a list of 12 positive qualities of effective clinical educators: (1) approachable, (2) good communicator, (3) in control, (4) knowledgeable, (5) self-aware, (6) self-confident, (7) concerned about patient

Clinical Educator Behaviors	Score
Communication Skills	
Makes himself or herself understood	
Provides useful feedback	
Is an active listener	
Provides positive feedback on performance	
Communicates in a nonthreatening manner	
Openly and honestly reveals perceptions of the student	
Provides timely feedback	
Is open to discussing issues with the student	
Teaches in an interactive way, encouraging dialogue	
Provides feedback in private	
Interpersonal Skills	
Establishes an environment in which the learner feels comfortable	
Provides support for the student's concerns, frustrations, and anxieties	
Empathizes with the student	
Demonstrates a genuine concern for clients	
Introduces the student to others as a professional	
Demonstrates a positive regard for the student as a person	
Professional Behavior Skills	
Demonstrates occupational therapy skills with confidence	
Exhibits professional behavior as part of the health care team	
Demonstrates a systematic approach to problem-solving	
Is able to explain occupational therapy treatment concepts to others	
Explains the goal of occupational therapy evaluation to others	
Demonstrates the role of occupational therapy in health care	

(Continued)

FIGURE 4.1. Characteristics of effective clinical educators: A self-assessment tool.

Clinical Educator Behaviors	Score
Serves as an appropriate role model	
Manages his or her own time well	
Demonstrates leadership among peers	

Teaching Skills

Allows the student progressive independence, as appropriate	
Is available to the student	
Makes the formal evaluation a constructive process	
Makes effective learning experiences out of situations that arise	
Plans effective learning experiences for students	
Provides a variety of clients for the student to learn from	
Questions and coaches the student in a way that helps him or her learn best	
Points out discrepancies in the student's performance	
Provides unique learning experiences	
Demonstrates the relationship between academic and clinical knowledge	
Is accurate in documenting student's performance evaluation	
Helps the student define specific learning objectives for fieldwork	
Observes student performance in a discreet manner	
Schedules regular supervision meetings with the student	
Plans learning experiences for the student before he or she arrives	
Manages the student's time well to ensure that learning objectives are met	
Is timely in documenting the student's written evaluations	
Is perceived as a consistent extension of the academic program	

Note. Scale: 1 = *I am not at all comfortable with this behavior, it is difficult for me, I lack experience;* 2 = *I am some-what comfortable with this behavior, I have limited experience;* 3 = *I am comfortable with this behavior, I have some experience;* 4 = *I am very comfortable with this behavior, I have a great deal of experience.*

Source: Adapted from Emery, M., Effectiveness of the clinical instructor: Students' perspectives. *Physical Therapy, 64,* 1984, 1079–1083, with permission of the American Physical Therapy Association. This material is copyrighted, and any further reproduction or distribution is prohibited.

FIGURE 4.1. Characteristics of effective clinical educators: A self-assessment tool *(Cont.).*

care, (8) interested in the learning process, (9) good role model, (10) competent, (11) enthusiastic, and (12) organized. All three groups of respondents ranked the first two items—approachable and a good communicator—as the two highest attributes. The rankings of academic faculty (which in the article were called "tutors," as in British custom) and clinical educators differed, perhaps a result of the separation between academia and clinical practice. Previous studies had examined only the differences between clinical educators and students. The author's conclusions were that both the academic faculty and clinical educators are "vying for the hearts and minds of the students" (Cross, 1995, p. 512). She felt that perhaps these two groups represent two different traditions: the higher education tradition and the health services tradition. This dissociation certainly sounds very familiar to those in academia and practice in the United States who discuss the academic–practice divide.

In a more recent survey, Bennett (2003) asked practicing physical therapists to reflect on their clinical education experiences. Bennett identified a comprehensive list of 54 abilities and qualities of effective clinical instructors and organized them into five categories (p. 434):

1. *Teaching and learning approach:* approachability, enthusiasm, desire to facilitate learning, ability to inspire motivation, good listening skills, integrity, patience, and sense of humor
2. *Management and organization of placement:* ability to provide timetable for learner, good time management skills, ability to delegate, provision of a stress-free team environment
3. *Continuing professional development in teaching and learning:* good communication skills, engagement in dialogue with university faculty, solid knowledge, awareness of research linking theory and practice, and knowledge of students' curriculum
4. *Facilitation of learning:* generosity in sharing knowledge with learner, skill in asking questions to promote learning, reflective practice, ability to discuss clinical reasoning, participation as a team player, and good problem-solving skills
5. *Teaching and learning process:* ability to give honest and constructive feedback, establishment of learning objectives, skill in providing learning opportunities, ability to make student feel valued, encouragement of hands-on experience, good teaching skills, ability to provide a varied caseload, and adaptability to students' varied personalities.

The results of Bennett's survey reinforced the findings of Cross's (1995) earlier study. Respondents ranked most highly those clinical educators who were interested in the learning process, rating the top three characteristics as approachability, enthusiasm, and good communication skills.

Clinical Supervision in Occupational Therapy

Christie, Joyce, and Moeller (1985) published the first study in occupational therapy to distinguish characteristics of effective and ineffective supervisors. They mailed open-ended surveys to fieldwork supervisors around the country; 188 were returned from a variety of practice settings. In addition, 127 student questionnaires were collected from 38 different occupational therapy education programs. Results were examined separately and then compared: "Supervisors and students concurred in their responses; both consistently liked certain behaviors with certain attitudes to distinguish the effective from the ineffective supervisor" (p. 677).

Effective supervisors were found to demonstrate good interpersonal and communication skills, active listening, openness, and honesty; to provide feedback that was timely, constructive, consistent, constructive, and growth producing; to be able to adapt their supervisory approach; to be flexible, open-minded, and available; to be competent as a clinician and as an educator; to have good role modeling, organizational, and teaching skills; to be supportive, empathetic, and nondefensive; to show concern for the student's growth; to be committed to the supervisory role; to be sensitive to students' needs; and to be patient, objective, and enthusiastic.

In contrast, students and supervisors listed the following characteristics as indicative of ineffective supervisors: poor interpersonal and communication skills; inability to effectively provide feedback; unwillingness to remain available to supervisees; lack of clinical experience or supervisory skills; rigidity; attitudes stifling creativity, originality, and independent problem-solving; controlling, dominating, smothering, and restrictive attitudes; and lack of support, caring, or concern for students.

Christie and colleagues (1985) found that occupational therapy students who experienced personal emotional responses during fieldwork, such as depression, anxiety, and stress, decided not to pursue practice in that particular area. They noted, "If students do not feel they can discuss such problems with a supportive supervisor, their unresolved feelings may contribute to the future avoidance of a particular area of practice or compromise the future therapist's ability to provide optimal patient care" (p. 677).

Christie and colleagues (1985) further examined the supervisors' level of education and training and the primary problems they faced in providing fieldwork supervision. Seventy-eight percent lacked formalized training, but 64% felt prepared to assume the fieldwork supervisor role because of their own clinical expertise, motivation, and interest in supervising students. The supervisors identified the problems and needs of dealing with students' affective and attitudinal behaviors, their own poor time management skills, lack of supervisory problem-solving skills, and inadequate academic and theoretical preparation of students. In conclusion, the authors noted that fieldwork supervisors are a primary influence in students' selection of a practice area and that students' experiences with supervision distinguish positive from negative fieldwork experiences.

Kautzmann (1990) reported findings from another study that surveyed fieldwork supervisors' attitudes and values around teaching. Seventy-five practitioners from around the country ranked (from most important to least important) 13 principles of adult learning (Knowles, 1980b) as follows (Kautzmann, 1990, p. 837):

1. Need for a thorough orientation
2. Value of incorporating students' interests, skills, and experience
3. Respect for learners' feelings and ideas
4. Ability to adapt teaching to each student's level
5. Need to be a resource person and provide feedback
6. Need to function as a team member
7. Need for students to identify their own learning needs
8. Involvement of students in evaluating their performance
9. Collaborative development of learning objectives
10. Importance of adjusting instruction to students' learning style
11. Importance of assessing students' knowledge at start of fieldwork
12. Desirability of involving students in planning their own learning
13. Collaborative development of evaluation criteria.

The author concluded that fieldwork supervisors' greatest need is for information about how to individualize fieldwork and how to plan, implement, and evaluate students' learning experiences.

Hummell (1997) reviewed Christie and colleagues' (1985) and Kautzmann's (1990) research and surveyed students in an educational program in Australia to determine if the previous findings were relevant. Hummell also sought to determine if students' responses were different based on what year in the professional program they were in. The results of this qualitative research design confirmed the previous results. Students characterized the following supervisory behaviors as most effective (pp. 150–152):

• Being approachable
• Being easy to talk to
• Listening to students' opinions and ideas
• Being interested in students
• Showing respect
• Providing support when needed

- Encouraging empathy and rapport
- Understanding the student's role
- Being aware of students' needs, fears, and concerns
- Being flexible and enthusiastic
- Appreciating and being sensitive to the individuality of each student
- Providing clear expectations
- Engaging in discussions with students about clinical issues
- Grading students according to students' individual skill levels
- Facilitating active student participation
- Encouraging students' self-direction and development of new competencies
- Offering supportive criticism of students' abilities
- Providing clear and tactful feedback to enhance student's strengths and limit their weaknesses.

Hummel (1990) concluded that

> effective fieldwork supervisors were viewed as collaborators and facilitators of learning who were willing to share their knowledge, provide clear expectations, grade tasks for students, encourage students to articulate their rationales for interventions, and were knowledgeable about the university course. They were perceived as skilled clinicians who behaved in a professional manner and provided clear, accurate and constructive feedback and evaluation in a supportive manner. An ineffective supervisor lacked all such skills and qualities. (p. 154)

 Learning Activities

1. Figure 4.1 lists the 43 behaviors Emery (1984) cited as being characteristic of clinical educators. Use this list as a self-assessment, and rate your own behavior on each item using the following 4-point scale: 1 = *I am not at all comfortable with this behavior, it is difficult for me, I lack experience;* 2 = *I am somewhat comfortable with this behavior, I have limited experience;* 3 = *I am comfortable with this behavior, I have some experience;* 4 = *I am very comfortable with this behavior, I have a great deal of experience.*

2. Based on your self-assessment, what do you perceive as your strengths as a clinical educator? What do you need to learn to increase your level of competence and confidence? Consider using those areas you scored low in to help set your professional development goals.

3. Describe an effective learning experience that you had either as the supervisor of a fieldwork student or while you were a fieldwork student. Then, describe a situation that resulted in a negative or ineffective learning experience for a fieldwork student or for you as a student.

4. Campbell (2000) created the list of effective supervisory behaviors and helpful personality characteristics in Exhibit 4.1 (to follow). Select 8 to 10 supervisory behaviors that you feel are the most important, and identify some that are not so important. Now do the same with the list of personality characteristics.

5. From your own experiences as a supervisee, make a list of at least 10 qualities you feel are descriptive of effective clinical supervisors. Then list some descriptors of ineffective supervisors.

6. Looking back on your experience as a student, what did you need most from your supervisor? If you are now a practitioner, what do you want most from clinical supervision?

EXHIBIT 4.1. Effective Supervisory Behaviors and Helpful Personality Characteristics

Effective Supervisory Behaviors	Helpful Personality Characteristics
Clarifies expectations	Sense of humor
Identifies style of supervision	Integrity
Maintains consistent boundaries	People orientation
Has knowledge of theory and practice	Trustworthiness
Teaches practical skills	Honesty
Provides frequent supervision	Tenacity
Encourages exploration of new ideas	Openness
Fosters autonomy	Flexibility
Models appropriate ethical behavior	Competence
Has a personalized therapeutic style	Credibility
Is personally and professionally mature	Consideration
Is willing to serve as a role model	Respectfulness
Perceives growth as an ongoing process	Understanding
Assesses the learning needs of the student	Sensitivity
Provides constructive feedback	Objectivity
Is invested in the student's development	Tact
Creates a relaxed learning environment	Genuineness
Cares about the well-being of others	Curiosity
Has the ability to be present and immediate	Intelligence
Has an awareness of his or her own personal power	Warmth
Has the courage to expose his or her own vulnerabilities	Supportiveness
Can acknowledge making mistakes	Tolerance
Is nonauthoritarian and nonthreatening	Availability
Accepts and celebrates diversity	Congruence
Is able to communicate effectively	Encouragement
Is aware of his or her own limitations and strengths	Easy-going attitude
Is willing to negotiate	Approachability
Works collaboratively	Creativity

Source: Copyright © 2000. *Becoming an effective supervisor: A workbook for counselors and psychotherapists,* by Jane Campbell. Reproduced by permission of Routledge, a division of Taylor & Francis Group.

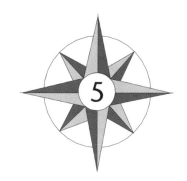

Theories About Learning

If in an educational situation an adult's experience is ignored, not valued, it is not just the experience that is being rejected, it is the person.

(Knowles, 1983, p. 61)

Clinical supervision has three functions—educational, monitoring, and supportive. In considering the educational function, one also must consider learning theories. Occupational therapy practitioners make a commitment to lifelong learning. As Knowles (1983) suggested, people bring their life experiences with them to any new teaching or learning situation. These experiences shape their attitudes and motivation to embark on new learning. This chapter reviews the major adult learning theories most relevant to clinical supervision in occupational therapy, as well as types of learning, domains of learning, learning styles, and learning processes. For the purposes of this book, I define each learning principle as follows:

- *Learning theories* are conceptual descriptions that explain how adults learn.
- *Learning styles* are the particular ways in which adults go about learning new things. Learning styles are unique to an individual, although some commonalities exist among them.
- *Learning types* are constructs, or ways of categorizing learning styles that are closely aligned with personality types.
- *Learning domains* are ways of classifying learning in a system (e.g., learning that is primarily focused on learning facts is classified as the cognitive domain).
- *Learning processes* are the manner in which new material is learned (e.g., deep or superficial learning).

Overview of Adult Learning Principles

Fieldwork educators frequently supervise students with different levels of competencies. Even if fieldwork educators treat their students exactly the same, providing the same assignments and expectations, the students' grades may differ. Likewise, two therapists attending the same continuing education workshop may not get the same results. Part of the reason for these discrepancies can be explained by adult learning theories. Different individuals learn in different ways. Familiarity with adult learning theories can help fieldwork educators assess students' learning styles, assess their own teaching style, design an educational experience most appropriate for each student's learning needs, and explain differences in student outcomes.

Andragogy is the "art and science of how adults learn, as contrasted to pedagogy, the art and science of helping children learn" (Knowles, 1980a, p. 43). Pedagogy is a more teacher-centered approach, whereas andragogy is a more learner-centered approach. One of the main differences between the two is the motivation to learn. With children, that motivation is external—parents and schools tell children they must go to school. But adults learn based on what's best for them, as an answer to the question "What's in it for me?" Adults' definition of who they are is phrased in terms of their accumulated and unique experiences:

> Asked who they are, adults are likely to define themselves in terms of their occupation, work history, where they have traveled, what education and experience has enabled them to do, and what their achievements have been. An adult is what he or she has done. (Cross et al., 2006, p. 71)

How do adults learn? Malcolm Knowles, one of the leading authorities on adult education and training, and his colleagues Edward Holton and Richard Swanson (2005, p. 3) identified six core adult learning principles:

1. *The learner's need to know*—Adults need to know why they are learning what they are learning. Specifically, they want to know three things: how the learning will be conducted, the content of the learning, and the rationale for why the learning is important.
2. *Self-concept of the learner*—Knowles et al. (2005) observed that "adults, and adults in the United States in particular, have a self-concept of being independent. In fact, it is having the freedom to choose their learning strategy that is critical" (p. 189). Thus, adults' self-concept is shaped by their responsibility for their own life decisions (autonomy) and their capability in and preference for self-directed learning.
3. *Prior experience of the learner*—Individuals have had different life experiences. This variability provides a rich resource for learning, but it also creates certain biases and negative effects. Because people's life experiences define who they are, learning provides the foundation for self-identity.
4. *Readiness to learn*—Adults are ready to learn when their lives create a need to know. This principle has two dimensions: the learner's need for assistance, which is related to level of competence in the subject and degree of dependence, and the amount

of support the learner needs from others during the learning process, which is influenced by the learner's commitment to the learning process and level of confidence in his or her ability to learn.

5. *Orientation to learning*—Adults are life-centered, task-centered, and problem-centered. They learn new knowledge best when the information is presented in real-life situations. This principle is closely related to educational theorist David Kolb's concept of experiential learning, which I cover later in this chapter.

6. *Motivation to learn*—Adults are motivated by external pressures, such as increased salaries, job promotions, or bigger houses, and by internal pressures, such as better quality of life and increased self-esteem, job satisfaction, or life balance. Research has repeatedly shown that in adults, internal pressures are stronger motivators (Knowles et al., 2005, p. 68).

Some of Knowles's (1980a) work has been criticized by other learning theorists, who feel that the Knowles principles of adult learning are the ideal, not the norm (e.g., Cross et al., 2006). Developmental psychologists such as William G. Perry, Jr. (1970) have conceptualized four stages that adult learners progress through:

1. *Dualism:* Learners at this stage recognize only two aspects to any given situation—right and wrong. Similarly, they feel that there can only be only one right answer to any question. Learners at this stage may view the educator as having all of the answers, and they are driven to know which answer the educator wants to hear. They need security and do best in situations in which the educator gives them the correct answers.

2. *Pluralism:* During this stage, learners begin to realize that there may be more than one answer to a question, and they begin to discover that the experts have multiple opinions. Learners find the variety of opinions confusing, but they begin to be able to express their own opinions.

3. *Relativism:* The confusion that learners experience during the preceding stage is replaced with acceptance as they acknowledge that there are multiple opinions. They experience a corresponding sense of freedom as they are able to admit that they are different from others.

4. *Commitment:* Learners experience a sense of security in this stage that is characterized by the need to widen their perspective. They can tolerate the divergent opinions of others.

Adult Learning Theories

More than 60 distinct educational theories have been developed since the late 19th century. Many educational researchers have attempted to classify these theories into broad categories, but there is no agreement on these classifications. We discuss the learning theories most relevant to clinical supervision in this section. (See http://tip.psychology.org/ for more detailed descriptions of each of the learning theories.)

Cognitive Theories

Cognitive theorists such as philosopher and psychologist Jean Piaget, psychologist Jerome S. Bruner, and educational psychologist Robert Mills Gagné focused their research on how people think and how they search for meaning. Cognitive theories emphasize principles that address perceptual features (e.g., sequencing, direction, figure–ground discrimination, relatedness of concepts), the organization of knowledge (from simple to complex or part–whole learning), culturally relative learning, cognitive feedback, and goal setting. Piaget's (1970) stages of development were based on the mental and cognitive abilities of children from infancy through adolescence. Bruner (1961) defined learning in terms of intellectual growth, development of competencies, and development of one's potential. Gagne (1965) proposed a hierarchy of learning from simple to complex; he suggested that students must master lower-level abilities before they can move on to higher-order ones. Gagne's hierarchy of learning included four stages: (a) facts, (b) concepts, (c) principles, and (d) problem-solving (cited in Knowles et al., 2005).

Behavioral Theories

Behaviorists, such as American psychologist Burrhus Frederic Skinner (1954) and Russian physiologist, psychologist, and physician Ivan Petrovich Pavlov (1927), focused their research on how learning occurred and cited the major components of learning as being a stimulus, a response, and a reinforcer. Behavioral learning theories focus on the effect of feedback on learning, the importance of task repetition in changing behavior, and the importance of active learning, or learning by doing, over passive learning. Successful learning outcomes result when correct behavior is rewarded until the learner consistently demonstrates the changed behavior. Clinical supervisors are responsible for shaping and changing students' behaviors by reinforcing or rewarding desired behaviors and negatively reinforcing or "punishing" undesirable behaviors.

Gestalt Theories

Gestalt theories are classified as field theories, meaning that "the total pattern or field of forces, stimuli, or events determine learning" (Knowles et al., 2005,

p. 29). People react to complex patterns of stimuli in organized wholes, rather than as disconnected parts. Four "laws" explain how people organize their perceptual fields (Knowles et al., 2005):

1. The *law of proximity* states that people view the parts of the stimuli that are closest together as a group.
2. The *law of similarity and familiarity* states that people group together objects with similar forms, shapes, colors, or sizes.
3. The *law of closure* explains people's need to complete the incomplete or to fill in the missing gaps in information.
4. The *law of continuation* states that people's perceptions are driven by organization; thus, if one sees three sides of a square or part of a circle, one recognizes it as a square or as a circle.

Humanistic Theories

The humanistic psychologists, most notably the approach's founders Carl Rogers (1969) and Abraham Maslow (1970), recognized that learning involves emotional as well as cognitive aspects. The thoughts and feelings of the learner are driven by his or her search for meaning. Maslow is best remembered for his theory of the hierarchy of human needs, in which basic physiological needs such as food, water, and sleep form the base of a triangle, with successively higher layers representing safety needs, the need to belong, and self-actualization at the top. The implication for learning is that people cannot learn when their basic needs are not met. Maslow stated,

> Growth takes place when the next step forward is subjectively more delightful, more joyous, more intrinsically satisfying than the previous gratification with which we have become familiar and even bored; the only way we can ever know that it is right for us is that it feels better subjectively than any alternative. The new experience validates itself rather than by any outside criterion. (quoted in Knowles et al., 2005, pp. 47–48)

Rogers (1969) did not think that a person can be taught anything directly; he believed that teachers are really just facilitators of learning. His emphasis on the personal learner–teacher relationship led him to identify three attitudes or qualities of effective facilitators: (a) realness or genuineness; (b) nonpossessive caring, prizing, trust, and respect; and (c) empathic understanding and sensitive and accurate listening. Rogers also identified the following 10 principles of learning (quoted in Rose & Best, 2005, pp. 126–127):

1. Humans have a natural potential for learning; it is the facilitator who sets the mood and climate of the learning experience or class.

2. Learning is effective when it is perceived as being relevant to the learner; the facilitator can help this along by clarifying the purposes of the class or learning experience.

3. Learning that results in a change in self-concept will be threatening to the learner, who will tend to resist.

4. Learning that is perceived by the learner to be threatening to him- or herself can be facilitated or encouraged in a supportive environment.

5. Opportunities for learning that may lead to fundamental changes in oneself can only occur if the threats to the learner are minimized.

6. Significant learning occurs by doing.

7. Learning is best facilitated when the learner is responsible for the learning.

8. Learning that is of a lasting, sustained nature involves feelings as well as the intellect.

9. Self-evaluation facilitates interdependence, creativity, and self-reliance much better than external evaluation.

10. The most socially useful learning is learning the process of learning, a continuing openness to experience, and incorporating oneself into the change process.

Clinical supervisors can apply these theories from humanistic psychology by

- Focusing on developing a supportive learning environment,
- Recognizing their role as effective facilitators of students' learning,
- Encouraging students to be more autonomous and to take responsibility for their own learning, and
- Remembering the negative impact that stress and anxiety have on the learning process.

Constructivism

The primary idea behind constructivism is that learners construct their own knowledge based on what they already know. This concept implies an active rather than passive learning process in which the learners make their own decisions about when and how to modify their existing knowledge base (Kaufman, 2003). Constructivism has important implications for clinical education; as in humanistic theory, teachers are viewed as facilitators of learning. Teachers can design learning experiences in which inconsistencies in knowledge will become evident to learners, leading them to explore further knowledge. Active problem-solving and group-learning activities are ideal ways to actively engage students in the acquisition of new knowledge, but learners need time to examine new experiences and construct new knowledge.

Learning Styles

People have different ways of processing, internalizing, and responding to the challenge of new learning, and these ways are referred to as *learning styles*. This section summarizes several models of assessing learning styles. Familiarity with learning styles can help clinical supervisors design learning activities in ways that support and maximize learning.

Kolb's Experiential Learning Cycle

Kolb's experiential learning cycle involves a cyclical process of perceiving and processing learning. Successful learning involves moving through the entire cycle of concrete experiencing, reflective observing, abstract conceptualizing, and active experimenting, but each person develops an individual preference for one of these elements. Kolb developed the Learning Style Inventory (LSI), which measures how an individual emphasizes one of the four learning modes (cited in Cara & MacRae, 2005). The LSI can help fieldwork educators assess the learning styles of themselves or others; it is inexpensive and widely available in print and online scoring versions. The four learning modes are as follows:

1. *Concrete experience* (CE) involves learning by feeling and by involving oneself fully and openly in a new situation.
2. *Reflective observation* (RO) involves learning by reflecting on and observing experiences from different perspectives or looking for meaning.
3. *Abstract conceptualization* (AC) involves learning by thinking or creating concepts by integrating observations, logically analyzing ideas, or planning systematically.
4. *Active experimentation* (AE) involves learning by doing, taking risks, and using hypotheses to guide and create new experiences.

Kolb described four learning styles that are based on combinations of modes (cited in Cara & MacRae, 2005):

1. *Divergers* (RO/CE) use reflective observation and concrete experience to learn. They perceive information concretely and then reflect on it. These people are generally imaginative, are good at generating multiple ideas in brainstorming sessions, can view situations from multiple perspectives, are open minded, and understand people.
2. *Assimilators* (AC/RO) enjoy taking in abstract ideas and concepts and then reflecting on them. They take a "watch-and-think" approach, are generally more interested in concepts than in people, are good at planning and creating theoretical models, are patient, and are less concerned with the practical application of theory.

63

3. *Convergers* (AC/AE) like to define and solve problems; they take in information abstractly and actively process it through experimentation and deductive reasoning. They are generally logical, are less emotional, are less interested in people, and are good at applying ideas in a practical manner.

4. *Accommodators* (AE/CE) take in concrete information and process it actively through doing. They like getting things done, take risks, initiate, can quickly adapt to circumstances, are intuitive, and are action oriented.

Psychologist Peter Honey and management trainer and developer Alan Mumford developed another learning styles questionnaire based on Kolb's experiential learning cycle. This questionnaire results in one of four learning styles (Cross et al., 2006):

1. *Activists* like to engage fully in the here and now; they are open minded and not skeptical of new ideas. They are enthusiastic about new things and enjoy brainstorming. Activists are bored during long-term implementation phases, are outgoing, and actively involve themselves in groups of people. They are positive about learning, dislike planning and/or preparation, do not enjoy reflecting on things, and can be very domineering in groups.

2. *Reflectors* are thoughtful and enjoy standing back to reflect. They like to observe things from a variety of perspectives and collect data and observations before reaching conclusions. They are cautious and thorough during planning stages, enjoy watching people in action, listen well to others, and maintain a low profile in groups. Reflectors prefer to take a back-seat approach during meetings, are generally reluctant to take risks, and are less likely to seize opportunities as they present themselves.

3. *Theorists* are good at identifying causal relationships, and they think problems through in a step-by-step manner. They like to analyze situations and appear detached and analytical to others. Theorist set high standards for themselves, are less interested in the emotional aspects of things, and may complicate issues, leading to a slowness to take action.

4. *Pragmatists* enjoy trying out new ideas in the real world, and they like to experiment. They tend to get impatient with lengthy discussions, because they want to act quickly. Pragmatists are positive and anticipate improvement; they like learning that is relevant to them and their situations and dislike an emphasis on theoretical concepts.

Myers–Briggs Type Inventory

The Myers–Briggs Type Inventory (MBTI) is based on Swiss psychology pioneer Carl Jung's (1969) archetype model and categorizes the ways individuals receive, store, and process information. There are four pairs of differences:

1. *Focus of interest:* On this continuum, people focus either on the outer world of people (extroversion, E) or on the inner world of ideas (introversion, I).
2. *Information gathering:* This continuum refers to the way individuals gather knowledge, by relying either on facts and ideas (sensing, S) or on intuition to understand meaning (intuiting, N).
3. *Involvement with information:* Individuals either focus on their subjective experiences (feeling, F) or rely on an objective analysis (thinking, T).
4. *Information management:* In managing information, people either attempt to regulate and control (judging, J) or look to experience life and adapt to it (perceiving, P).

An individual's scores on the MBTI reflect each of the four continuums, and the scores determine which of 16 personality types (e.g., ESFJ, INTP) the person fits. Kitzrow (2001) researched the use of the MBTI in clinical supervision and made recommendations for supervisors based on their predominant style. Table 5.1 summarizes the characteristics and strengths of each personality dimension and recommendations for skills to work on (Bernard & Goodyear, 2004).

Dunn and Dunn's Learning Styles Model

Educational researchers Rita and Kenneth Dunn (e.g., Dunn, 2000; Dunn & Dunn, 1998) developed a learning styles model in which they identified 21 elements of stimuli in five categories that influence a learner's ability to process new information:

1. *Environmental stimuli* include sound, light, temperature, and seating arrangement.
2. *Emotional stimuli* include motivation, persistence, responsibility, and structure.
3. *Sociological stimuli* include the preference for learning alone or with peers, in dyads, in teams, with adults of similar ages, or in varied social contexts.
4. *Physical stimuli* include perceptual stimuli (auditory, visual, tactile, and kinesthetic), intake stimuli (eating vs. not eating), peak energy levels according to time of day, and mobility (sitting still vs. moving around).

TABLE 5.1. Characteristics and Strengths of Supervisor Personality Dimensions and Suggestions for Skills on Which to Work

Supervisor's Personality Type	Natural Characteristics and Strengths	Supervision Skills on Which to Work
Extraverted	Takes an active approach Helps students explore a wide range of interests and issues Is open, expressive, and energetic Processes information and solves problems externally through interaction and dialogue	Help students explore issues and cases in depth Slow down and allow time for reflection and processing Talk less and listen more
Introverted	Allows time to process information internally Helps students explore issues and cases in depth Takes a reflective approach Is skilled at one-on-one communication	Help students focus on action as well as reflection Talk more and try to be more open and expressive
Sensing	Focuses on dealing with present issues and concerns Is good at details and facts Helps students identify practical, step-by-step action plans Is practical and realistic	Be open to varied approaches rather than just tried-and-true methods Encourage students to use intuition and imagination as well as facts Step back to consider the big picture, patterns, and new possibilities
Intuitive	Encourages students to use and trust intuition and imagination Enjoys abstract thinking, theories, and identifying patterns and meanings Focuses on dealing with potential issues and concerns that may arise in the future Is skilled at helping students see the big picture and possibilities	Be more attentive to facts, details, and issues that need immediate attention Integrate theories with practical applications

(Continued)

TABLE 5.1. Characteristics and Strengths of Supervisor Personality Dimensions and Suggestions for Skills on Which to Work *(Cont.)*

Supervisor's Personality Type	Natural Characteristics and Strengths	Supervision Skills on Which to Work
Thinking	Is good at solving complex problems Is intellectually challenging Is logical Uses an objective, analytical approach	Balance theory with concrete examples and practical approaches Be more subjective; take feelings and values, as well as logic and analysis, into consideration Moderate the tendency to be overly challenging and critical Remember to give positive feedback
Feeling	Is empathetic, supportive, and collaborative Is good at facilitating the growth and development of others Seeks harmony and avoids conflict	Address conflicts and problems that arise in supervisory relationship and help students address issues with clients Be more objective; take analysis and logic, as well as feelings and values, into consideration Provide challenges as well as support
Judging	Attends to details, schedules, and deadlines Helps students plan and implement therapeutic goals in a structured manner Is structured and organized; dislikes disruption in routine or last-minute changes	Be more flexible, spontaneous, and open to innovative approaches Focus on process, not just on goals or deadlines Remember to give positive feedback
Perceiving	May overlook schedules and deadlines Is open to new and innovative approaches; encourages students to try new approaches Is spontaneous, flexible, and tolerant; adapts to last-minute changes or crisis well Tends to procrastinate and put off tasks and decisions	Be aware of tendency to procrastinate and to miss deadlines or details Keep up with paperwork, reading, case notes, and viewing of tapes Conduct supervisory sessions punctually and in a structured manner Help students develop goals and structured treatment plans

Source: Adapted from Kitzrow, M. (2001). A model of supervisory style based on psychological type. *The Clinical Supervisor, 20*(2), 133–146. Reprinted with permission from the Haworth Press © 2001.

5. *Psychological stimuli* involve such preferences as global versus analytical, hemisphericity (being left or right brained), and impulsive or reflective.

Types of Learning

Experiential Learning

As its name implies, *experiential learning* refers to learning that occurs within the demands of everyday life rather than formal learning in a classroom. The focus is on practice, not theory. Experiential learning that occurs within informal, everyday contexts also has been called *situated cognition* or *professional knowledge* (Cross et al., 2006). Kolb (1984) is best known for his work on the experiential learning cycle; the four elements of learning are represented in Figure 5.1.

Kolb's is not a static learning model but rather a dynamic one, where the learner enters at any stage in the model and progress through the cycle. The learner has to move through all four stages for learning to be fully integrated. The four parts of the reflective learning cycle are as follows:

1. *Concrete experience* refers to being fully involved in a learning experience in the here and now.

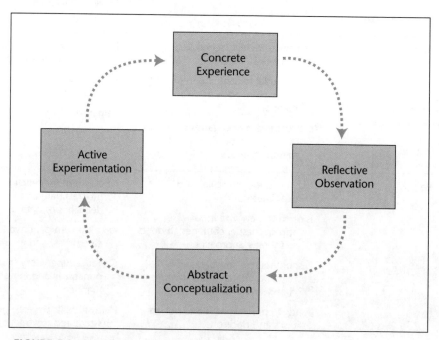

FIGURE 5.1. Experimental learning cycle.

2. *Reflective observation* has to do with reflecting on or critically thinking about the learning experience in which one has been engaged.

3. *Abstract conceptualization* refers to making connections between what one has just learned and prior learning and/or experience in an attempt to create patterns and form theories or hypotheses about those patterns.

4. *Active experimentation* occurs when the learner tests out new ideas, bringing theory and practice together to make decisions and solve problems.

Reflective Practice

Reflective practice will be explored in more depth in Chapter 12. Philosopher, researcher, and theorist Donald A. Schön, who is credited with being a leader in the concept of reflective practice, theorized that classroom learning has limitations in everyday practice. Schön conceptualized two types of reflective practice. The first, *reflection-in-action,* involves the application of current and past experiences to unfamiliar events as they are occurring. The second, *reflection-on-action,* happens later, after the event is over. It is characterized by thinking back on what happened and what contributed to the event, evaluating whether the actions taken were appropriate, and examining how a similar situation might be handled in the future—a kind of "Monday-morning quarterbacking" analysis. Clinical educators can encourage this type of reflective practice by assigning journals, debriefing learners after critical incidents, and seeking feedback from learners on a regular basis (Kaufman, 2003).

Problem-Based Learning

Problem-based learning (PBL) is a curricular strategy based on constructivist theories in which learning occurs in small groups of students discussing real-life clinical problems. Students' prior knowledge is integrated as they work through the clinical cases, and extensive discussion with peers integrates new knowledge. Clinical educators who have been trained in a PBL model should tailor learning assignments and perhaps undergo specialized training in the use of PBL as a continuing education model in the clinic.

Clinical Skills Learning

Many skills used in clinical occupational therapy practice are manual skills in that they involve physical handling of patients and/or equipment. Learning manual skills requires a different format, because these skills require hands-on practice, ideally first in the classroom and then in the clinic. The multiple components involved in learning manual skills include the following:

- Defining what the skill is, how and when it is used, contraindications for use, and any safety precautions;
- Demonstrating the skill, which involves the instructor first demonstrating the skill as it should be correctly performed;
- Practicing the skill, often repeatedly on peers, until it becomes a habitual practice;
- Receiving feedback from peers and the instructor about performance and modifying Behavior based on feedback; and
- Transferring the skill to a new setting, usually the clinic, with patients.

Collaborative Learning

Collaborative learning is an extension of constructivist theory in which groups of learners collaborate, or work cooperatively, to construct new knowledge. This type of learning can involve groups of students working together under one fieldwork supervisor, groups of two or more members of the same profession, or teams of members from different professions. Collaborative learning has been cited in the literature repeatedly as an effective learning model in which the clinical educator is viewed not as the expert with all the answers but rather as a co-learner engaged in an active learning process.

Domains of Learning

Educational psychologist Benjamin Bloom (1956) made significant contributions to the classification of educational objectives and the theory of mastery learning, including developing a way to categorize the domains of learning that became known as Bloom's taxonomy. The three domains separate the various types of knowledge and, within each domain, present multiple levels of increasing knowledge. The taxonomy can be very helpful to clinical educators in designing behavioral objectives for learning that demonstrate progression.

Cognitive Domain

The cognitive domain involves knowledge, thinking, and the development of intellectual skills. Its levels distinguish lower-level thinking from higher-level thinking, suggesting a way that people learn about information. The levels from lowest to highest are as follows:

- *Knowledge* refers to the observation and recall of data or information, such as dates, events, or places; of major ideas; and of subject matter.
- *Comprehension* involves understanding information, grasping meaning, translating knowledge into a new context, interpreting facts, comparing and contrasting, and stating a problem in one's own terms.

- *Application* refers to the use of information, methods, concepts, and theories in new situations and the solving of problems using knowledge or skills.
- *Analysis* is concerned with seeing patterns or the organization of parts, recognizing hidden meanings, identifying components, and distinguishing facts from inferences.
- *Synthesis* refers to the ability to generalize information based on given facts, to use old ideas to create new ideas, to relate knowledge from several areas, to predict or draw conclusions, to create new meanings or structure, and to put together the parts to form a whole.
- *Evaluation* is concerned with comparing and discriminating between ideas, assessing the values of theories, making choices, verifying the value of evidence, recognizing subjectivity, and making judgments about the value of ideas or materials.

Table 5.2 lists the levels in the cognitive domain of Bloom's taxonomy, with the corresponding action verbs associated with each level.

TABLE 5.2. Bloom's Taxonomy: Cognitive Domain

Knowledge	Comprehension	Application	Analysis	Synthesis	Evaluation
Cite	Compute	Apply	Analyze	Arrange	Appraise
Count	Convert	Calculate	Appraise	Assemble	Assess
Define	Describe	Discover	Calculate	Collect	Choose
Draw	Discuss	Dramatize	Categorize	Compose	Compare
Know	Explain	Employ	Compare	Construct	Criticize
List	Identify	Examine	Contrast	Create	Estimate
Match	Locate	Illustrate	Debate	Design	Evaluate
Name	Paraphrase	Interpret	Diagram	Formulate	Judge
Quote	Report	Operate	Differentiate	Integrate	Measure
Recite	Restate	Practice	Examine	Manage	Rank
Record	Review	Schedule	Infer	Organize	Rate
Relate	Summarize	Sketch	Inventory	Plan	Revise
Repeat	Tell	Solve	Question	Prescribe	Score
Underline	Translate	Use	Test	Propose	Select

Source: Adapted from p. 99 of Rose, M., & Best, D. (2005). *Transforming practice through clinical education, professional supervision, and mentoring.* New York: Elsevier. Reprinted with permission from Elsevier.

Affective Domain

The affective domain focuses on the ways people deal with things emotionally, including their attitudes, feelings, values, and interests. Within it are five levels:

1. *Receiving* refers to attending to an issue, being aware, and being willing to hear.
2. *Responding* implies active participation of the learner through his or her reactions to the issue at hand.
3. *Valuing* involves the relative importance that the learner attaches to an object or behavior based on internal judgments or values.
4. *Organizing* involves prioritizing issues in terms of their importance after deciding their value and emphasizes comparing, relating, and synthesizing values.
5. *Characterizing* (sometimes referred to as *internalizing values*) refers to the issue's inherent value to the learner. At this level the behavior is pervasive, consistent, and predictable; it has become characteristic of the learner.

The verbs used with the affective domain are listed in Table 5.3.

Psychomotor Domain

The psychomotor domain focuses on learning that involves physical action, movement, physical handling, and motor skills. There are seven levels within this domain:

TABLE 5.3. Bloom's Taxonomy: Affective Domain

Receiving	Responding	Valuing	Organizing	Characterizing
Attend	Complete	Believe	Display	Act
Choose	Comply	Defend	Favor	Influence
Accept	Answer	Accept	Codify	Internalize
Develop	Cooperate	Devote	Judge	Perform
Name	Discuss	Influence	Order	Qualify
Realize	Examine	Prefer	Organize	Revise
Receive	Obey	Pursue	Relate	Serve
Recognize	Observe	Seek	Systematize	Solve
Ask	Behave	Balance	Discriminate	Verify
Reply	Respond	Value	Weigh	

Note: Original table based on format from table in Rose, M., & Best, D. (2005). *Transforming practice through clinical education, professional supervision, and mentoring.* New York: Elsevier.

1. *Perception* involves awareness of and ability to use sensory cues to guide motor activities.
2. *Set* refers to the readiness to act and includes physical, mental, and emotional sets, or dispositions, that determine a person's response to different situations.
3. *Guided response* refers to the early stages of learning a complex skill in which the learner uses imitation and trial-and-error learning. Repeated practice leads to improvement in performance.
4. *Mechanism* is the middle stage of learning a complex skill; some of the responses have become habitual and are performed with proficiency.
5. *Complex overt response* refers to proficiency in complex motor acts that are now performed quickly, accurately, and in a coordinated manner. The learner is able to perform a skill without hesitation in an almost automatic manner.
6. *Adaptation* implies that the learner now possesses well-developed skills and can adapt them to different situations based on the demands of the environment.
7. *Organization* means being able to create new patterns to fit different situations or problems.

Table 5.4 lists verbs associated with the psychomotor domain.

TABLE 5.4. Bloom's Taxonomy: Psychomotor Domain

Perception	Set	Guided Response	Mechanism	Complex Overt Response	Adaptation	Origination
Taste	Position	Imitate	Manipulate	Operate	Supply	Arrange
Touch	Prepare	Inject	Mix	Assemble	Adapt	Combine
Distinguish	Adjust	Copy	Adjust	Calibrate	Alter	Construct
Hear	Approach	Determine	Build	Coordinate	Build	Create
See	Locate	Discover	Illustrate	Demonstrate	Change	Design
Choose	Volunteer	Repeat	Set up	Mix	Revise	Initiate
Smell	Place	Duplicate	Indicate	Maintain	Develop	Produce

Note: Original table based on format from table in Rose, M., & Best, D. (2005). *Transforming practice through clinical education, professional supervision, and mentoring.* New York: Elsevier.

Learning Processes

The FAIR Approach

Hesketh and Laidlaw (2002a, 2002b) described a partnership model of controlling the learning process based on the following four principles:

1. *F*eedback that is constructive and frequent throughout the learning experience is most helpful to the learner. It encourages learners to self-assess and motivates them to address their deficiencies and learning needs.
2. *A*ctivities, and a wide variety of them, need to be provided that promote collaborative as well as self-directed learning. The assignment of activities promotes active learning rather than passive learning.
3. An *I*ndividualized approach that is responsive to each learner's needs, preferred learning style, and pace of learning is the most productive in encouraging learners to be responsible for their own learning. Learning contracts are an ideal method for promoting an individualized approach.
4. The *R*elevance of learning experiences to each learner is essential to the attainment of learning objectives. Learners are more motivated to learn when they perceive that the assignments are meaningful to their identified learning goals.

Levels of Learning

Entwistle (1987) described four approaches to learning (see also Wickham, 2005a):

1. The *deep approach* to learning is characterized by the learner's intention to understand the material to be studied and commitment to relate ideas to the new material, rework it, and use evidence to test it. Student who use this approach are often considered "model students"; in a practicing therapist, it is evidence of a "reflective practitioner."
2. The learner who adopts the *surface approach* intends simply to reproduce the material to be learned, as in rote learning or memorization. Resulting knowledge is context bound and difficult to apply in new situations.
3. Learners using the *strategic approach* attempt to find out exactly what is required of them, which may lead to either a surface or deep approach. The student picks up cues from the educator and wants to excel or please the educator.

4. The *apathetic approach* to learning is almost a non-approach; there is little, if any, intention on the part of the learner. Students who use this approach are often considered "clueless" and show a lack of direction or interest in the subject.

Clinical supervisors need to encourage learners to adopt the deep approach, in which the learner is able to grasp concepts. The following teaching approaches facilitate deeper levels of learning:

- Involve learners in the selection of subjects to be studied and learning methods to increase internal motivation.
- Design learning activities that facilitate active rather than passive learning.
- Discuss ideas and concepts as a group; interaction with others promotes reflection on learning and helps learners test new concepts.
- Facilitate the integration of new knowledge into the learner's knowledge base.
- Use collaborative learning strategies with pairs or small groups of learners.
- Maximize the use of experiential learning activities.
- Generate real-life problem-solving situations for learners.

 Learning Activities

1. Think of a course or workshop you attended that provided you with a positive learning outcome. What factors promoted your ability to learn? List factors that were intrinsic to you, the learner; those that were related to what the instructor did well; and those that were related to the way the course was structured.

2. Identify a course or workshop that you are planning to take or wish to take in the future, and answer the following questions:

- Why do you want to take the course?
- What do you feel you will gain from taking the course?
- How you will prepare yourself for the course?
- What behaviors will you demonstrate during the course that will facilitate your learning?
- What aspects of the course are you looking forward to?

3. Think of a course or workshop that you have attended, and identify the factors that had a positive effect on your learning. Factors can include the structure of the learning, the supervisor's style, the environment, the pace, the feedback, or any other factors you wish to identify. Were there any negative factors?

4. Recall one of your own fieldwork or later clinical supervision experiences, and identify the factors that had positive and negative effects on your learning. Identify factors that had a negative impact on your learning.

5. Think of a time you had to teach someone else a skill. Describe the experience in terms of the skill, the skills you used in instructing the learner, and the outcomes. How effective was your teaching strategy, given the other person's learning style? Reflect on how you know the answer to this question.

6. What motivates you to perform at your best? Do you reward yourself after you've completed a learning task, and if so, how? Have you ever had to motivate someone else to learn to do something? How did you motivate that person?

7. Think of a time when someone asked you the question, "How do you know that?" How did you respond?

8. Review the list of characteristics associated with each of the learning styles identified in the Honey and Mumford's experiential model. Which of the attributes do you think describe you best? Do the same with Kolb's (1984) experiential learning cycle model. How do your attributes compare with those of students you are teaching or have taught?

9. Use Tables 5.1, 5.2, and 5.3 outlining Bloom's level-of-learning domains to help you write specific learning objectives for fieldwork supervision.

10. Think of a subject you have tried to master, course material you have tried to study, or a complex book you have tried to read for continuing education. For each of the stimulus preferences listed in Figure 5.2 (as follows), write down a description of the conditions you needed to learn best. For example, under the category of sound, do you learn best when it's quiet, do you need soft background noise, or do you study best when you blast loud music?

Stimulus Preference	Conditions You Need to Learn Best
Sound	
Light	
Temperature	
Seating arrangement	
Motivation	
Persistence	
Responsibility	
Structure	
Alone (self)	
In pairs (dyads)	
In small groups	
In teams	
With peers	
With teachers or tutors	
Auditory	
Visual	
Tactile	
Kinesthetic	
Time-of-day energy levels	
Intake (eating, drinking)	
Mobility (sitting still or moving)	
Hemisphericity (right-brain or left-brain orientation)	
Impulsive or reflective	
Global or analytic	

Source: Partial data from Dunn & Dunn, 1998.

FIGURE 5.2. Self-assessment using Dunn and Dunn learning style preferences.

11. In what ways do your own learning styles influence your teaching or supervisory style?

12. Do you think a supervisor's learning style should be the same as or different from that of supervisees?

13. Complete one of the learning inventories mentioned in this chapter to gain further insights.

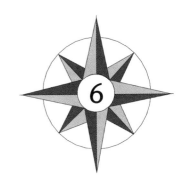

Assessing Readiness to Become a Clinical Supervisor or Fieldwork Educator

The move to a more student-centered view of learning has required a fundamental shift in the role of the teacher. No longer is the teacher seen predominantly as a dispenser of information or walking tape recorder but rather a facilitator or manager of students' learning. . . . The more responsibility given to the student, the greater the shift in the teacher role.
(Harden & Crosby, 2000, p. 339)

In Chapter 2, I reviewed the history of clinical supervision, noting that in its earliest beginnings, people who aspired to various professions learned their craft via the apprenticeship model: Novice learners worked directly under masters, watching how they worked and modeling their behavior based on their observations. When universities became the source of professional education, there was a shift to learning in the classroom and then going out into the real world to practice and apply that knowledge. Experienced professionals are given the responsibility to serve as teachers, guides, mentors, and evaluators of students, but in most professions, they have been given little or no formal education to guide their transition from the role of clinician to the role of clinical educator. How, then, do occupational therapists or occupational therapy assistants assess their readiness to assume the role of fieldwork educator or clinical supervisor?

Theories of Clinical Supervisor Development

Several theories have been proposed that address how practitioners move from being a clinician to being a teacher. One of the most widely cited is the Dreyfus model of skill acquisition, developed in 1980 by brothers Hubert and Stuart Dreyfus, a philosopher and an applied mathematician, respectively. They studied chess players, Air Force pilots, and Army tank drivers and commanders in examining how skills developed (Benner, 2004).

The resulting model is a developmental one that is influenced by experiential learning. This model formed the basis of a landmark study conducted by nurse Patricia Benner (1984) of nurses at varying levels of work experience. Her findings supported the Dreyfus model, articulating the same five stages of development:

1. *Novice:* Students in their first year of professional education are at the novice level of development. They have little, if any, experience with patient care, and their knowledge comes primarily from their instructors and texts. The novice's behavior is governed by rules, and novices need detailed, clear instructions.

2. *Advanced Beginner:* New graduates are usually advanced beginners. Although they still follow the rules, they are beginning to learn how to apply those rules in new situations. There is enormous pressure on them to perform well, which often leads to anxiety and fatigue. Advanced beginners rely heavily on feedback from colleagues, patients, and family members, and they still rely on textbooks for descriptions of patients' signs and symptoms because they have limited experience in viewing these firsthand.

3. *Competent:* Practitioners with 1 to 3 years of practice typically are in the competent category; they have a sense of mastery and can cope with most clinical situations. They plan their work tasks to increase efficiency and organization. They do not yet perform tasks with speed but are methodical in their performance. Clinicians at this stage are beginning to feel responsible for their own actions and often lose confidence in others, for which they sometimes compensate by studying from comprehensive textbooks.

4. *Proficient:* Clinicians who are proficient are both accountable and intuitive and no longer rely solely on book knowledge. Their performance is more consistent at this stage. They are able to view the big picture rather than just the individual parts. The anxiety that characterized the earlier stages has now been replaced by a sense of being at home in the clinical environment. Proficient practitioners can accommodate rapidly to variations in clinical conditions, because they have more clinical experience to draw on.

5. *Expert:* Expert clinicians are recognized for their practical wisdom. They are able to rapidly assess a situation and make decisions about how to proceed, and they are able to deal with the unexpected. As a result, they can manage complex clinical situations and recognize patterns or trends in service provision. They appear almost intuitive in their ability to assess a situation and know exactly how to proceed.

The Dreyfus model of skill acquisition can be applied to fieldwork education for occupational therapists. In the novice stage, the student has no experience with being an occupational therapist or with supervision. They may do well in the classroom, but they become frightened when they begin field-work and believe their knowledge to be insufficient. Their initial clinical experiences may be characterized by passive learning, observation of the fieldwork educator, and heavy reliance on their textbooks for the answers to clinical questions. In terms of clinical supervision, they have not learned yet what is required of a supervisee, and thus, they may need direction on how to best use supervision.

In the advanced beginner stage, the occupational therapist or occupational therapy assistant has just completed training and begun a first job. The first year of practice has a steep learning curve. A supervisor may no longer direct the practitioner's every task; feedback may be delayed, and supervision may be infrequent. Advanced beginners sometimes feel that they don't know enough to practice. Practitioners at this stage should obtain regular clinical supervision on their own if it is not provided at their place of employment; new graduates are frequently advised by their academic programs not to work in an independent practice setting the first year.

In the competent stage, practitioners have 1 to 3 years of experience and are beginning to feel comfortable with the realities of clinical practice. They are likely to be assigned their first fieldwork student at this stage, and they may feel a sense of panic at the prospect of teaching someone else. Unless they have had formal training in how to be a supervisor, they tend to imitate the supervisors they had as students. Many competent practitioners have worked in only one setting and thus may have limited knowledge of the variety and complexity of clinical conditions. They may be caught off guard by fieldwork students' questions but may feel that they must know more than their students.

During the proficient stage, the occupational therapist or occupational therapy assistant can view the entire clinical situation as a whole rather than as separate parts. They can improvise solutions when presented with unexpected situations. They may be promoted to fieldwork site supervisor, overseeing the supervision of multiple students and practitioners.

By the expert stage, occupational therapy practitioners have acquired practical wisdom; they know how to proceed in complex clinical situations almost intuitively. They might be promoted to a managerial role at this point, or they may venture into designing and implementing their own fieldwork program.

Lived Experience Model

Speech pathologist Lindy McAllister developed the lived experience model in 2001 based on qualitative research interviews with speech pathology clinical educators at varying levels of experience. Her analogy for becoming a clinical educator was "becoming comfortable in new shoes" (Higgs & McAllister, 2005, p. 159). She identified six dimensions in being a clinical educator (p. 156):

1. *Sense of self:* McAllister described a sense of self as a core phenomenon that includes not only self-awareness, self-acceptance, and sense of identity but also the extent to which the clinical educator seeks to control people, time, and events. Sense of self is an intrapersonal dimension.

2. *Sense of relationship with others:* This interpersonal dimension involves the clinical educator's ability to accurately perceive others as they are, to be more people oriented than self-absorbed, and to base practice on humanistic values. In occupational therapy, therapeutic use of self in working with clients reflects this dimension.

3. *Sense of being a clinical educator:* Being a clinical educator involves understanding the work environment in which one practices and fulfilling the dual responsibilities of caring for patients and simultaneously instructing students.

4. *Sense of agency:* "Refers to how people see themselves, the types of relationships they value, and how confident and competent they feel in being empowered to act within the context they are placed, including both situational constraints and opportunities available to them" (Higgs & McAllister, 2005, p. 164). McAllister used the metaphor of a juggler when describing this dimension; the clinical educator sets up an environment that both supports and challenges student learning.

5. *Seeking dynamic self-congruence:* Dynamic congruence involves clinical educators' trying to live out their values through the learning they facilitate in their students: "The aim is to seek congruence between one's evolving self-identity, planned actions, and actual behaviors and actions" (Higgs & McAllister, 2005, p. 164).

6. *Growth and development:* There is a developmental progression in becoming a clinical educator, from survival to complex maturity and from a focus on oneself to a focus on others. The goal is to achieve what Higgs, Titchen, and Neville described as "professional artistry—the meaningful expression of a uniquely individual view within a shared tradition" (quoted in Higgs & McAllister, 2005, p. 165). Clinicians who have achieved this goal have acquired the just-right blend of practice skills, practitioner qualities, and creativity in designing and implementing effective learning activities for students.

This model is not sequential but rather is complex and multidimensional and can serve as a self-assessment tool for clinicians aspiring to be fieldwork educators. In each dimension, the practitioner self-assesses where he or she is on a continuum and designs a professional development plan for increasing growth in each dimension. A professional development plan is a type of learning assessment and learning contract that provides a self-assessment of strengths for areas that need to be addressed, with stated learning objectives, methods, and time frames to accomplish them. It is similar to a treatment plan that an occupational therapist would devise for their clients. The last page of the AOTA *Self-Assessment Tool for Fieldwork Educator Competency* is a Professional Development Plan (Appendix D).

Role Competencies for Fieldwork Educators

The American Occupational Therapy Association (AOTA), through its Commission on Education (COE), has developed role competencies for fieldwork educators following the Standards for Continuing Competence (AOTA, 2005), reprinted in Appendix A. These competencies describe the values, knowledge, skills, and responsibilities that occupational therapists or occupational therapy assistants need to be successful in the role of fieldwork educator. Occupational therapy practitioners can use these standards, which are reflected in the following questions, to assess their own competency as a fieldwork educator.

Standard 1: Knowledge

In addition to being able to demonstrate knowledge of clinical practice, fieldwork educators have to be able to answer the following questions regarding knowledge about supervision:

- Do I know how to facilitate learning in students so that they achieve entry-level competency in a particular practice area by the end of the fieldwork experience?
- Do I know how to design learning activities and assignments that reflect the breadth and depth of the learning required of a competent entry-level practitioner?
- Do I understand what is involved in effective learning processes and techniques that support students' individual learning styles?
- Do I understand everything that is detailed in the contract signed by the university or college and the facility in which I work?
- Have I achieved competency in occupational therapy processes and supervision skills through continuing education, formal education, and/or self-study?
- Am I aware of the various standards, rules, and laws regarding the supervision of students that have been developed in my state, by accrediting bodies (e.g., the Joint Commission on the Accreditation of Healthcare Organizations or the Accreditation Council for Occupational Therapy Education [ACOTE]) and the facility I work for?

Standard 2: Clinical Reasoning

Clinical reasoning forms the foundation for clinical decision making in occupational therapy. In addition to meeting this standard for practice as an occupational therapist or occupational therapy assistant, the fieldwork educator needs to know the clinical reasoning involved in fieldwork supervision, as reflected in the following questions:

- Am I able to locate, read, effectively evaluate, and share new materials, literature, and educational materials about fieldwork education with colleagues and students that will encourage lifelong learning in future practitioners?
- Can I critically integrate and apply theory, literature, and research into practice at my fieldwork site?
- Have I read and understood, and am I able to critically evaluate, the components of the curriculum of the schools that send me fieldwork students as these components relate to best practice in fieldwork education?
- Am I able to evaluate the interpersonal dynamics at my fieldwork site among practitioners, clients, and students in order to resolve any conflicts that might develop? Can I create an action plan to remedy conflicts, and do I know when I need to notify the academic fieldwork coordinator of the school?

Standard 3: Interpersonal Skills

Being an occupational therapy practitioner means being able to develop professional relationships with others in the clinical practice setting. Fieldwork educators must likewise be able to answer affirmatively the following questions related to interpersonal skills:

- Do I project a positive image of my fieldwork site's program to the college or university that sends students?
- Do I demonstrate that I am competent and project a positive attitude toward practice and supervision so that fieldwork students will receive effective mentoring and guidance in their development of entry-level competencies?
- Can I effectively supervise fieldwork students on practice-related issues throughout their fieldwork experience?
- Am I able to mediate any interpersonal issues that may develop among students, clients, and other practitioners or staff?
- Do I consistently demonstrate cultural competence in my interactions with faculty, students, practitioners, and academic fieldwork coordinators from diverse backgrounds?

- Am I able to identify and communicate clearly to students their strengths and weaknesses in a respectful manner that facilitates their personal and professional growth?

Standard 4: Performance Skills

Occupational therapists and occupational therapy assistants must be able to demonstrate the expertise, attitudes, proficiencies, and abilities needed to perform skills and fulfill roles competently. Fieldwork educators need to be able to respond affirmatively to the following questions:

- Can I plan fieldwork experiences at my site that will prepare ethical and competent entry-level practitioners?
- Do I know how to develop site-specific objectives, course materials, and learning activities that will promote optimal learning in the students I supervise?
- Am I comfortable evaluating students' performance on specific learning objectives at midterm and final evaluations?
- Do I know how to design, implement, and maintain a system of documentation for all aspects of the fieldwork program, including evaluation of student performance, collaboration with the academic institution, contact with the academic fieldwork coordinator, and any other required documentation?

Standard 5: Ethical Reasoning

Occupational therapists and occupational therapy assistants must be able to identify, analyze, and clarify issues involving ethical dilemmas. As fieldwork educators, they need to be able to respond affirmatively to the following questions:

- Am I able to act as a role model for occupational therapy advocacy and as a change agent in a manner that is professional, culturally competent, and ethical?
- Can I clarify and analyze fieldwork issues within an ethical framework, leading to a positive and successful resolution?

Self-Assessment of Fieldwork Educator Competency

The Commission on Education Fieldwork Issues Committee designed a self-assessment instrument in 1997; it is longer and more detailed than the Role Competencies for Fieldwork Educators, but fieldwork educators can translate the information directly into a professional development plan. The tool addresses five areas of supervisory competencies to be self-evaluated on a continuum from low proficiency to high proficiency. The entire document is reprinted in Appendix G; the following subsections summarize the various fieldwork educator competencies.

Professional Practice Competencies

To be a fieldwork educator, the practitioner must have previously acquired competency in practice. To that end, one of the requirements established by ACOTE for becoming a fieldwork educator is 1 year of practice. The following questions can help practitioners assess their practice competencies:

- Do I use a systematic approach to client evaluation and treatment based on theory?
- Do I skillfully collect and analyze evaluation and treatment data?
- Do I consider performance contexts when I am designing a treatment plan for a client?
- Am I able to objectively define my client's strengths and weaknesses?
- Am I able to articulate the rationale, theory, and frame of reference behind my interventions with clients?
- Am I able to collaborate with individuals, colleagues, clients, families, and others in a way that demonstrates respect, sensitivity, and professional judgment?
- Do I work effectively with challenging situations, such as those involving cultural diversity, value differences, or personality conflicts?
- Can I effectively manage my daily clinical practice and prioritize issues as necessary?
- Am I aware of ethical, legal, and professional issues that influence my practice, such as confidentiality laws, reimbursement guidelines, and role delineation?
- Can I articulate the collaboration that exists between the occupational therapist and the occupational therapy assistant?
- Do I adhere to professional practice standards?
- Do I assume responsibility for pursuing continuing education to expand my knowledge and skills in accordance with the principles of lifelong learning?

Education Competencies

Education competencies are concerned with the fieldwork educator's ability to facilitate the development of professional skills in students. Practitioners who wish to supervise fieldwork students should be able to respond affirmatively to the following questions:

- Am I able to assess students' individual learning needs, both initially and throughout their fieldwork experience, on the basis of their academic preparation, life experiences, and performance?
- Do I know how to sequence learning activities to provide developmental progression as the student's abilities improve?

- Do I understand what is meant by student-centered learning, and am I able to facilitate that learning?
- Am I able to use planned and unplanned experiences to maximize students' opportunities for learning?
- Am I able to use more than one instructional strategy to facilitate students' learning, such as role modeling, cotreating, collaborative learning, videotaping, and so forth?
- Can I work effectively with all students, including those with physical and/or psychosocial disabilities and those of different ages, genders, educational levels, ethnicities, religions, and cultures?
- Do I feel comfortable guiding students in their integration of therapeutic concepts and skills? Can I ask students the right questions to elicit the clinical reasoning behind their selected treatments? Can I engage students in discussions about how their personal feelings and values interface with practice?
- Have I evaluated my own competencies as a fieldwork educator and created a fieldwork educator professional development plan?
- Can I identify and locate resources that will facilitate professional development in students and fieldwork educators?
- Am I able to provide students and other fieldwork educators with reference materials on fieldwork education such as books, articles, videotapes, and Internet resources?

Supervision Competencies

Supervision competencies focus on the fieldwork educator's abilities to monitor and guide students toward the achievement of entry-level practice competency. The following questions can help practitioners assess their level of competency in providing supervision:

- Can I clearly present to students the level of performance expected of them when they begin fieldwork and throughout the experience?
- Am I comfortable collaborating with students as they set learning goals, learning objectives, and performance expectations? Can I modify learning experiences based on this collaboration?
- Am I able to anticipate and prepare students for clinical situations that may be challenging?
- Do I provide learning activities to students that will provide the just-right challenge?
- Am I comfortable giving students prompt feedback that is direct, constructive, and specific? Am I equally comfortable giving positive and negative feedback to students?
- Am I able to give specific suggestions to students about ways they can improve their performance?

- Do I communicate effectively through verbal, nonverbal, and written communication?
- When there is conflict, am I able to initiate discussion with the individuals involved to resolve the conflict? Can I initiate conversation about difficult issues?
- Can I use a variety of supervisory approaches to facilitate student performance, such as support, confrontation, written feedback, or consultation with other supervisors?
- Am I able to elicit student feedback about the fieldwork experience? Can I get students to discuss their concerns? Am I able to respond to them effectively, even when the feedback or issues are difficult?
- Can I collaborate with the student and academic fieldwork coordinator when the student is having difficulty in order to identify and modify learning situations and activities?
- Am I able to act as a role model for professional behavior? Can I separate personal from professional issues? Can I address diversity issues in a culturally competent way? Can I use humor when and if appropriate?

Evaluation Competencies

Being a fieldwork educator involves the ability to evaluate student performance. The following questions address the specific competencies involved in evaluation:

- Do I review with students the evaluation tool that will be used to assess their performance on fieldwork at midterm and final evaluations?
- Am I able to assess student performance objectively through direct observation, discussion with the students, review of written work, or another format?
- Can I assess students' level of performance based on established entry-level competencies for the occupational therapist or occupational therapy assistant?
- Am I able to ask students questions that will lead them to engage in self-reflection and self-assessment during the evaluation process?
- Can I help students focus on their strengths and opportunities for growth during the evaluation process?
- Do I complete and distribute on time all required fieldwork evaluations?
- Am I able to help students view the evaluation process as a way to grow professionally and personally?
- Am I aware of students' legal and ethical rights in the fieldwork evaluation process with regard to due process, confidentiality, disability issues, and integrity?

Administrative Competencies

Fieldwork education involves numerous administrative tasks that the fieldwork educator needs to complete during fieldwork. The following questions address the administrative function:

- Am I able to communicate and collaborate with the various educational programs that send their fieldwork students to my site in such areas as scheduling, contracts, interviews, and requirements?
- Do I seek support from my administrator for the fieldwork program?
- Am I able to design and implement the fieldwork program in compliance with current AOTA policies and standards such as the *Code of Ethics, Standards for Practice, ACOTE Standards,* and *Role Competencies for Fieldwork Educators?*
- Can I provide assurance to schools and students that fieldwork staff are sensitive to diversity and cultural issues?
- Have I established the fieldwork site's policies and procedures in an organized way, such as providing a fieldwork manual and a weekly outline of student expectations or assignments?
- Am I able to write site-specific behavioral objectives for occupational therapist and occupational therapy assistant entry-level practice?
- Can I define the roles and responsibilities of a fieldwork student at my site according to established agency, state, and national policies and guidelines?
- Am I able to provide a designated work area for students?
- Do I provide students with a complete orientation to the policies and procedures of the fieldwork site?
- Do I ensure that students are aware of and comply with the fieldwork site's mission, goals, philosophy, and standards?
- Do I submit all required paperwork to the school in a timely manner?
- Do I conduct ongoing evaluations of the fieldwork site and monitor changes in the program with student and staff input (primarily through AOTA's Student Evaluation of Fieldwork Experience and Fieldwork Data forms, found on the Fieldwork Education Web page at www.aota.org/nonmembers/area13/links/link07.asp)?
- Fieldwork educators can use the responses to these questions to identify their areas of strength and areas they need to develop. These insights can be used in creating a professional development plan with specific goals, time frames, and learning strategies.

Learning Activities

1. Create a supervision resume (Campbell, 2000, p. 245) to identify your preparation for the supervisory role. Start with your experience as a supervisee. List the fieldwork experiences you had—the settings, populations, duration of placement, tasks, and assignments. Was a particular style of supervision used (e.g., one-on-one, one-on-two, two-on-one, group, collaborative). Describe each of your supervisors' styles, techniques, supervisory models, and methods used. What evaluation methods did your supervisors use? What kind of feedback did you receive, and in what format? Next, list any experience you have had providing peer supervision and any other experience with being a supervisor or a supervisee outside of fieldwork. Finally, summarize your strengths as a clinical supervisor.

2. Identify what you believe to be the pros and cons of being a clinical supervisor or fieldwork educator. What makes you want to provide clinical supervision or fieldwork education?

3. Imagine an ideal fieldwork student. What traits and characteristics would he or she possess? Consider the following:

- Age
- Gender
- Educational level
- Ethnicity
- Religion
- Learning style
- Learning goals
- Level of maturity
- Physical characteristics (e.g., height, weight)
- Health status
- Prior experience
- Level of competence
- Personality
- Leisure interests
- Level of independence
- Sense of humor.

How do you think the presence or absence of these characteristics would affect your ability to supervise a student? In what ways is your ideal student similar to you? Using the same list, create a description of a student you would have difficulty supervising. How would you proceed with supervising your least-preferred type of student—what would you have to change to work effectively with this student?

4. Campbell (2000) identified 10 steps* toward building one's own model of supervision. Read through each of these steps, and answer the questions:

- *Step 1.* Identify your philosophy of change. How do you feel that people change?
- *Step 2.* Identify goals for supervision. What needs to be accomplished during the student's fieldwork experience? What does your supervisee need?
- *Step 3.* Define specific competency areas for supervision. What are the competencies that the supervisee needs to meet? What knowledge does he or she need? What skills must he or she be able to demonstrate?
- *Step 4.* Identify the expectations for supervisees at each developmental level. Can you identify expectations for each week of the fieldwork experience? What is the beginning expectation? The expectation at midterm evaluation? At final examination?
- *Step 5.* Assess the learning needs and developmental level of the supervisee. What are his or her skills and abilities? Life experiences? Academic preparation?
- *Step 6.* Identify the developmental level of yourself as the supervisor. How will you change the supervision you provide as the supervisee changes and grows?
- *Step 7.* Identify your preferred style of supervision. What methods do you feel most comfortable using?
- *Step 8.* Identify any environmental or contextual factors that may influence supervision. Are there any constraints that may have a negative impact on supervision, such as time, caseload, or an off-site supervisor?
- *Step 9.* Identify the nature and stage of the supervisory relationship. Is this the beginning, midpoint, or end? Is this an easy or conflicted relationship? Are there power or control issues to be addressed?
- *Step 10.* Identify the knowledge, skills, methods, and techniques that you need to develop or acquire to provide effective supervision. Can you identify a supervisor or mentor who can help you with this? (pp. 252–253)

---

*Copyright © 2000 from *Becoming an effective supervisor: A workbook for counselors and psychotherapists,* by June Campbell. Reproduced with permission of Routledge, a division of Taylor & Francis Group.

5. Supervisors tend to imitate the way they were treated as students. As clinical education experts Jane Westberg and Hillard Jason (1993) pointed out, "When trying to understand and analyze abstract ideas, most of us reflect on and make connections to our own experiences" (p. 23). Think about your own learning experiences, and respond to each of these questions (quoted from Westberg & Jason, 1993):

- Did my supervisors create an atmosphere of trust so that I could be open and honest in discussing issues with them?
- Did they create an environment that encouraged students to develop trusting relationships with each other?
- At the start of each of my fieldwork experiences, did my supervisors explain to me the goals and expectations that I was to accomplish by the end of the learning experience?
- Did my clinical supervisors assess my learning needs and learning style during my fieldwork experiences, and if so, how did they do that?
- Was I encouraged to develop my own learning goals for the fieldwork experience?
- Did my fieldwork supervisors collaborate with me in developing learning contracts that included learning activities, goals, and strategies?
- Did I receive enough feedback from my supervisors about my work? How was this feedback provided to me? Was I encouraged in any way to self-evaluate my work?
- If I was with other students during fieldwork, were we encouraged to provide feedback to each other?
- Was I treated as an active partner in the fieldwork experience?
- Did my supervisors facilitate collaboration between students, or was there competitiveness between us?
- Was I given the message, directly or indirectly, that students could and should contribute to each other's learning?

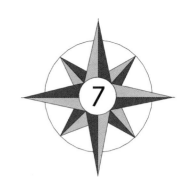

Assessing the Effectiveness of Clinical Supervision

Being a quality clinical educator is about taking a good look at ourselves.

(Rose & Best, 2005, p. 47)

When he was mayor of New York City, Ed Koch frequently would ask people, "How am I doing?" This question is precisely the focus of this chapter. How do fieldwork educators and clinical supervisors know whether or not they are providing effective guidance to their supervisees? What methods can they use to assess their performance as a supervisor on an ongoing basis? For fieldwork educators, the student evaluation of fieldwork experience provides feedback regarding the clinical education experience. There are at least two problems with this type of evaluation, however. First, the feedback comes at the end of the fieldwork experience, when it is too late to change anything. Second, students often report that they find it difficult to be candid in providing feedback to the fieldwork educator on an evaluation form, particularly if the experience was lacking in some way. This chapter explores some other ways for supervisors to assess their effectiveness.

Fieldwork Experience Assessment Tool

The Fieldwork Experience Assessment Tool (FEAT), developed by the Fieldwork Research Team in 1998, is reproduced in its entirety in Appendix C. The instrument is intended to facilitate a discussion between the fieldwork educator and the student about the three key components in fieldwork—the environment, the student, and the fieldwork educator. Ideally, it is used around the midpoint of a student's fieldwork experience so that if areas of concern are identified, changes can be made. Each item on the FEAT is scored on a continuum from *limited* through *excessive,* with *just-right challenge* being in the middle. The section of the FEAT that focuses on the fieldwork educator is an ideal way for educators to get some feedback on their effectiveness. The following questions reflect items from the FEAT that address the supervisor's effectiveness:

- Do you appear to like teaching and supervising students?
- Do you invest time in student learning?
- Do you display enthusiasm around students? Do you appear to enjoy the mental challenge of answering student questions?

- Are you available and accessible? Do you make time for regularly scheduled supervision sessions, or are you so busy that the student feels guilty about asking questions?
- Do you provide support to the student? Are you patient? Do you convey a positive and caring attitude toward the student? Do you encourage questions? Is the student encouraged to develop his or her own individual style?
- Are you an open and accepting supervisor? Are you able to use alternative supervisory or teaching methods? Are you open to student requests? Is your communication with students open?
- Do you organize information that you present to students? Do you have written learning objectives?
- Do you engage the student in dialogue about treatment?
- Are you able to structure supervision based on the student's needs?
- Can you identify strategies for helping the student adjust to the demands of the treatment environment?
- Do you expose the student to increasingly difficult or challenging cases as his or her skills increase?
- Are you able to provide the just-right challenge to the student as he or she progresses by reducing the amount of direction you give, asking probing questions, and allowing increased independence?
- Are you aware of the student's learning style, and do you modify your teaching accordingly?
- Do you promote independence in the student, encouraging him or her to use trial and error when appropriate?
- Are you able to provide the student with timely feedback that supports his or her growth?
- Can you balance positive and negative feedback?
- Are you able to guide the student's thinking?
- Can you promote the student's clinical reasoning skills?
- Do you regularly share your resources and knowledge with the student?
- Are you able to include the student as part of the treatment team?
- Do you provide role modeling for the student? Does he or she see you treating patients? Do you set a good example of professional behavior?
- Do you exhibit an enthusiasm for occupational therapy?
- Do you come across as a "real" person to the student?
- Do you demonstrate to the student that you value and engage in life-long learning?

Asking yourself the above questions is a good start in evaluating your effectiveness as a supervisor, but to obtain true feedback, you must ask students for feedback—"How am I doing?" You may think you're providing the just-right challenge to your students, but unless you ask them, you won't know for sure. Chapter 10 discusses ways to support students in providing honest feedback.

Performance of Students and Supervisees

Although formal evaluations are valuable, effective clinical supervisors are able to gauge their effectiveness on the basis of how well their students are doing in meeting their performance expectations. Postman and Weingartner (1969) described the "good teacher" as one who helps students achieve certain behavioral changes:

> the frequency with which they ask questions; the increase in the relevance and cogency of their questions; the frequency and conviction of their challenges to assertions made by other students or teachers or textbooks; the relevance and clarity of the standards on which they base their challenges; their willingness to suspend judgments when they have insufficient data; their willingness to modify or otherwise change their position when data warrant such change; the increase in their skill in observing, classifying, generalizing, etc.; the increase in their tolerance for diverse answers; their ability to apply generalizations, attitudes, and information to novel situations. (quoted in Westberg & Jason, 1993, p. 356)

Peer Review

Obtaining feedback from colleagues about your supervisory effectiveness is another form of assessment. There are many ways to do obtain input from your peers. One of the easiest ways to begin the journey of becoming a clinical supervisor is to jointly supervise a fieldwork student with another, more experienced colleague. Before the student arrives, agree with your peer on what each of you will be responsible for and what your roles will be; if this negotiation does not take place beforehand, the student may be caught in the middle between two opposing voices.

Another way to obtain feedback from peers is to videotape or audiotape your supervisory sessions—with your student's consent, of course. Videotaping is a powerful method of getting feedback: You will be able to see yourself as others see you, and your colleague can provide guidance and suggestions for ways to improve supervisory sessions.

A third way to engage in peer review is to form a supervision group of several colleagues who all have fieldwork students. Group sessions can be designed with a facilitator who has experience in clinical supervision, or the group members can facilitate their own inquiry.

Suggestions for Improving Your Effectiveness as a Clinical Educator

Westberg and Jason (1993, pp. 364–369) provided several suggestions of ways for clinical educators to improve their teaching effectiveness. The commitment to lifelong learning is not limited to clinical practice; for clinicians who are regularly involved in providing supervision, this commitment includes learning about teaching and supervising.

Periodically, review your own learning goals and objectives. What skill areas did you identify as needing further development on the professional development plan you developed in Chapter 6? Have you met the goals you established within the time frame you identified? If you have, what is the next learning goal you want to establish?

Make it a regular practice to inquire of your supervisees whether they're getting what they need from you. This inquiry can be helpful to both of you, and it encourages learners to be self-reflective, identifying what works for them and what does not. Sometimes students are caught off guard when their supervisor asks them to identify what else they need. This question may raise their anxiety level, and they may respond superficially and quickly with "Everything's fine." You have to dig deeper with open-ended, probing questions and then pause, waiting patiently while they think before responding.

After you have completed a midterm or final fieldwork performance evaluation on a student, take time to reflect on the progress the student has made. Then ask yourself what you did that contributed to the learner's meeting the expectations. What supervisory strategies or assignments did you use that worked well? What did not work so well? The student's success is, in part, your success.

Written feedback can be particularly helpful, but sometimes existing forms do not capture the feedback you are seeking. Feel free to experiment with creating your own forms for supervisees to complete. Perhaps you tried something new with a particular student and want to know whether it worked. You can create a form tailored to your methods and goals.

Invite trusted colleagues to provide you with feedback. Ask a peer to sit in on a supervision session with the purpose of giving you feedback. Or create a peer supervision group in which you and several colleagues can review supervisory strategies together in a trusting environment.

Enroll in workshops, or take courses on clinical supervision. If you can't find any offered by occupational therapists, consider taking one offered by another discipline such as physical therapy, social work, or nursing.

Find a mentor whom you can trust and who will guide you on your journey to excellence in clinical supervision. Consider being a mentor to someone more junior than yourself; it is often by teaching someone else that professionals accomplish their best learning. A mentor with experience in teaching and clinical supervision will be the most useful.

Invite the academic fieldwork coordinator to come and speak to you and your colleagues about best practice in fieldwork education. Many fieldwork consortia around the country offer continuing education workshops for fieldwork educators; consult the AOTA Web site for a listing of those consortia and contact information.

Create a library at your site that includes professional development material related to clinical supervision and fieldwork education. Many books are available on the subject and are included in an annotated bibliography at the end of this book. If your facility has a medical library, or if you have access to a local college or university library, use it to search for articles on clinical education, fieldwork, clinical supervision, learning, and other useful topics. A great deal of literature on clinical supervision is available on the Internet, so you can also use a search engine to find articles. Some of the journals that I have found helpful for educational and supervisor issues are

- *Journal of Physical Therapy Education*
- *Medical Teacher*
- *Learning in Health and Social Care*
- *Nurse Educator*
- *The Clinical Supervisor*
- *Counselor Education & Supervision*
- *Medical Education*
- *Academic Medicine*
- *Journal of Nursing Education*
- *Journal of Allied Health*
- *Internet Journal of Allied Health Sciences and Practice.*

Finally, as Westberg and Jason (1993) have pointed out,

Be patient with yourself. The more you know about effective teaching, the more challenging you are likely to realize it is. Give yourself time. Take risks, even though taking risks can involve going through periods of feeling functionally grotesque. Be patient with your self. And most of all—*have fun!"* (p. 369)

Learning Activities

1. Westberg and Jason (1993, pp. 370–371) developed the Supervisor Self-Assessment. Read each of the statements in Figure 7.1 and rate yourself on each item using the following scale: A = *always,* B = *most of the time,* C = *sometimes,* and D = *never.* Identify your strengths and areas where you have room for improvement.

2. Westberg and Jason (1993, pp. 372–373) developed a modified version of the Supervisor Self-Assessment for learners to fill out. Figure 7.2 is an adaptation of their evaluation form. Read each of the statements, and rate your ability to provide each skill area to supervisees, using the following scale: A = *always,* B = *most of the time,* C = *sometimes,* and D = *never.*

Statement	Score
1. I help supervisees assess their strengths at the beginning of the fieldwork experience.	
2. I develop a relationship with supervisees based on mutual trust and respect.	
3. I help supervisees develop their own learning goals and objectives.	
4. I provide opportunities for supervisees to practice the skills they are learning.	
5. I give clear explanations to supervisees of assigned tasks and check to make sure that they understand.	
6. I encourage supervisees to ask questions.	
7. I listen more than I speak.	
8. I encourage supervisees to self-evaluate their own performance.	
9. I provide regular feedback (positive and negative) to supervisees that is constructive.	
10. I provide a summary of performance to supervisees at the end of their fieldwork experience.	
11. I treat my supervisees in a supportive manner, expressing concern for their well-being.	
12. I encourage supervisees to be active partners with me in the learning process, collaborating to construct new knowledge.	
13. I provide supervisees with an effective role model for quality patient care.	
14. I enjoy teaching.	
15. I enjoy learning.	

Note. Use the following scores: A = *always,* B = *most of the time,* C = *sometimes,* and D = *never.*

Source: Westberg, J., & Jason, H. (1993). *Collaborative clinical education: The foundation for effective health care* (pp. 370–371). New York, NY: Springer. Reproduced with the permission of Springer Publishing Company, LLC, New York, NY, 10036.

FIGURE 7.1. Supervisor self-assessment.

Statement	Score
1. My supervisor helped me identify my strengths.	
2. My supervisor was someone I could trust and be honest with.	
3. My supervisor helped me develop learning goals and objectives.	
4. My supervisor gave me opportunities to practice the skills I was learning.	
5. My supervisor asked questions that made me think.	
6. My supervisor gave clear explanations when teaching me something new or assigning me a task.	
7. My supervisor encouraged me to ask questions.	
8. My supervisor listened attentively to what I had to say.	
9. My supervisor encouraged me to self-evaluate my own performance.	
10. My supervisor provided constructive feedback, both positive and negative, throughout my fieldwork.	
11. My supervisor provided me with a summary of my performance at the midpoint of fieldwork and at the end.	
12. My supervisor treated me with concern and respect.	
13. My supervisor invited and encouraged me to be an active partner in the learning process, collaborating on goals and assignments.	
14. My supervisor effectively modeled patient care.	
15. My supervisor appeared to really enjoy the teaching process.	
16. My supervisor was committed to and appeared to enjoy lifelong learning.	

Note. Use the following scores: A = *always,* B = *most of the time,* C = *sometimes,* and D = *never.*

Source: Westberg, J., & Jason, H. (1993). *Collaborative clinical education: The foundation for effective health care* (pp. 372–373). New York, NY: Springer. Reproduced with the permission of Springer Publishing Company, LLC, New York, NY, 10036.

FIGURE 7.2. Supervisor assessment for learners.

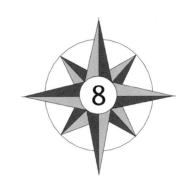

Cultural Competencies in Clinical Supervision

When two people meet in supervision . . . there is a negotiation that always happens. First, similarities are assessed, then dissimilarities. Color might be one . . . being from the same region might be another . . . having parents with similar emphases on education might be yet another. We then look to see how many of those dissimilarities can be bridged. The greater the effectiveness we have in bridging those dissimilarities, the greater the multicultural competence we have in supervision.

(Hird, Cavalieri, Dulko, Felice, & Ho, 2001, p. 117)

This chapter explores the influence of culture on clinical supervision in field-work and in practice. Diversity in the United States is increasing and is projected to continue to increase:

> Nearly 50% of the U.S. population will consist of ethnic minorities by 2050: Native Americans, Alaska Natives, Asians, Pacific Islanders, African Americans, Hispanics, and Latinos are expected to increase from 25% of the U.S. population in 1990 to 32% by 2010 and 48% by 2050. By 2080, for the first time in U.S. history, minority subgroups will comprise most of the U.S. population and are predicted to account for 55.6% of the total population. (Ekelman, Bello-Haas, Bazyk, & Bazyk, 2003, p. 131)

Supervisors need to be aware of the many possible differences between themselves and their supervisees. These differences may be in age, gender, religious beliefs, race, socioeconomic status, ethnicity, language or dialect, level of education, disability, sexual preferences, and worldview. According to Campbell (2000),

> It is not enough, however, for supervisors to be aware of, and sensitive to, how beliefs and attitudes about differences in people might affect their relationship with the supervisee. The effective supervisor must be able to respond to these differences. (p. 175)

Multicultural Competency in Supervision

Multicultural competency has been defined as a

> therapist's awareness of assumptions about human behavior, values, biases, preconceived notions, personal limitations, understanding the worldview of the culturally different client without negative judgments; and developing and practicing appropriate, relevant, and sensitive intervention strategies and skills in working with culturally different clients. (Sue, Arredondo, & McDavis, 1992, p. 481)

Multicultural competency includes attitudes, beliefs, knowledge, and skills. It is important for supervisors to define culture broadly "to include within-group demographic variables (e.g., age, sex, and place of residence), status variables (e.g., social, educational, and economic), and affiliations (formal and informal), as well as ethnographic variables such as nationality, ethnicity, language, and religion" (Pederson, 2000, p. 36).

Being culturally competent is not a state one achieves but rather a dynamic process that evolves over time; it involves "acceptance and respect for differences, continuing self-assessment regarding culture, vigilance toward the dynamics of differences, ongoing expansion of cultural knowledge and resources, and adaptations to services" (Ekelman et al., 2003, p. 132).

In the literature on multicultural and transcultural supervision, several studies have been reported that have implications for occupational therapy fieldwork supervision. One found that a large majority of supervisors in the field of counseling stated that they had never had a course on culture and that many of their supervisees had had more training in this area than their supervisors (Constantine, Warren, & Mivile, 2005). The authors also found that, in addition, the majority of therapists and their supervisees were White but their client caseloads were much more diverse.

A study by physical therapy educator Rick Ladyshewsky (1996) looked at the experiences of Asian students in a physical therapy training program in Australia. He found that some skills that educators value in students, such as self-directedness, assertiveness, and problem-solving ability, were unique to students who had been educated in Western educational programs. In Asian countries, students are raised to have respect for their teachers, in the same way that they are raised to have respect for their elders. The Asian students in this study believed that expressing views in the presence of a teacher who has more experience is disrespectful. Asian students also had difficulty self-evaluating their performance; one student commented, "Divulging negative aspects of your performance is something your elders would punish you for. . . . It is unusual to be encouraged to express your weaknesses. To praise yourself is not encouraged—it is important to be humble" (Ladyshewsky, 1996, p. 4).

Ladyshewsky (1996) also examined communication patterns, such as wait time between questions and answers, word selection, and communication style. Any of these can cause difficulty for students who are trying to communicate in a language that is not their primary one, as well as for supervisors with expectations and biases:

> Clinical instructors and academic programs need to improve their understanding of cross cultural supervision issues. Understanding the background culture of the student as well as the issues related to cross cultural supervision will make the learning experience more productive for all concerned. Again, one must be careful about generalizing and stereotyping. (p. 7)

Racial Identity Theory, Worldview, and Acculturation

An important construct in exploring cultural competence is *racial identity theory*, which involves individuals' psychological processes involving perceptions of power differentiated by race. This theory is grounded in racial identity schemata defined as "the dynamic cognitive, emotional and behavioral processes that govern a person's interpretation of racial information in her or his interpersonal environments" (Helms, 1995, p. 184). Helms and Cook (1999) theorized that the racial identity development process for White people comprises six stages, from first recognizing their false sense of racial superiority to eventually adopting a nonracist identity. Their model strongly supports the assertion that courses on culture must have students examine their own racial identity and worldviews before examining differences and similarities between and among other cultures.

Psychologists Carol Falender and Edward Shafranske (2004) suggested broadening the categories that need to be considered when exploring a person's worldview to include factors such as the following:

- Optimism and pessimism
- Traditional beliefs
- Attitude toward the present
- Social relations
- Time
- One's relationship with nature and living in harmony with nature
- Values (e.g., competition versus cooperation, emotional restraint versus expressiveness)

- Guiding beliefs (e.g., independence versus interdependence, control and dominance versus harmony and deference)
- Epistemology (e.g., cognitive versus affective or combined)
- Logic (reasoning process)
- Nature of reality (e.g., objective material versus subjective, spiritual versus material)
- One's concept of self. Also, direct attention to spirituality and religion should be highlighted. (p. 127)

Another important issue that has emerged in the supervision literature is the role of acculturation in international students. *Acculturation* refers to the adaptive process of changing behavior in response to a new culture. The length of time students have lived in the United States and the degree to which they have adapted to a Western worldview determine the extent of acculturation and of its influence on the supervisory relationship:

> International students in the early stages of the acculturation process may have more difficulties developing an alliance with their supervisors, may feel more uncertainty about the supervisory relationship, and may experience more role ambiguity than students who are more acculturated. (Nilsson & Anderson, 2004, p. 307)

Psychologists Johanna Nilsson and Mary Anderson suggested that supervisors need to discuss with supervisees from other cultures how emotions are expressed in their culture, how relationships are formed and sustained, views of mental illness, and what constitutes healthy behavior. Although self-disclosure is commonplace in the United States, it is not universally valued; people from other cultures may view self-disclosure as invasive or socially inappropriate. Nilsson and Anderson emphasized that

> the goal of supervision with international students is not to have them acculturate to the U.S. culture at the expense of their own culture. Given that 57% of these students planned to return to their country of origin, a more appropriate goal would be to assist them in becoming bicultural, and thus helping them function effectively as counselors in two cultures. (p. 311).

Importance of Multicultural Competency in Clinical Supervision

The role of cultural competence may be even more critical in clinical supervision than in direct practice. In supervision, the supervisor is responsible not only for the supervisee but also for the welfare of the clients whom the supervisee treats. Priest (1994) suggested that a supervisor must move through six stages to achieve multicultural competency in supervision:

1. In the first stage, the supervisor is in denial about cultural differences that may affect the supervisory relationship.
2. In the second stage, the supervisor admits that there are some cultural differences but does not know how to address them.
3. In the third stage, the supervisor begins to address cultural issues by identifying the similarities and differences between himself or herself and the supervisee.
4. In the fourth stage, the supervisor figures out where and how he or she fits into the cultural framework.
5. In the fifth stage, the supervisor begins to appreciate the unique aspects of the supervisee's culture.
6. In the sixth stage, the supervisor begins to translate and integrate this new insight into the practice of supervision.

Students who perform well in the classroom but then experience difficulties in the clinical education environment may be having problems with communication. Clouten, Homma, and Shimada (2006) highlighted the importance of conversational language skills to the success of clinical experiences:

> Delays in conversation can be interpreted as a lack of interest or a lack of knowledge when they are the result of time taken to process information, translate, and prepare a response. Students may also experience difficulty with sentence construction and word selection, resulting in overuse of some words and simple but abrupt sentences. (p. 4)

Self-Assessment of Multicultural Competency

Supervisors are responsible for ensuring that cultural factors contribute to, rather than detract from, the student's fieldwork experience. Psychologist Pamela Hays (2001) proposed an acronym to assist clinicians in exploring and addressing the multiple aspects of cultural competence. Each letter in the acronym ADDRESSING represents an aspect of culture that therapists and supervisors must consider:

A—age and generational influences
D—developmental problem
D—disability
R—religion and spiritual orientation
E—ethnicity
S—socioeconomic status
S—sexual orientation
I—indigenous heritage
N—national origin
G—gender.

The author suggested that after examining all of these aspects, therapists should also consider the role of privilege, culture, and personal values in their work with supervisees and clients.

Fieldwork educators are responsible for developing multicultural competence. Being aware of students' cultural background is not sufficient; fieldwork educators must be able to respond to the cultural issues that are present in the supervisory relationship and adapt their supervisory methods as necessary. Fieldwork supervisors should be especially alert to cultural issues when they are younger than their students, are the opposite gender, have a different sexual orientation, practice another religion, have only a bachelor's degree, or have a disability, to name just a few potential differences. They must be prepared to understand how these differences affect how they evaluate each student. They also must understand how these differences account for communication difficulties and consider any cultural biases that may affect their expectations of the supervisee. They must be prepared to use other methods for evaluating a student when the usual ones they use fail. They must know how to ask questions that will lead to a greater understanding of cultural similarities and differences, resulting in a stronger supervisory relationship. Fieldwork educators can begin by reflecting on their own experiences as a student, recalling any differences that were present in their own supervisory relationships.

Several multicultural competency skill surveys have been developed that might be helpful for new fieldwork educators. One is the Multicultural Awareness, Knowledge, and Skills Survey (D'Andrea, Daniels, & Heck, 1991), a 60-item self-assessment survey. Another is the 42-item Abbreviated Multidimensional Acculturation Scale (Zea, Asner-Self, Birman, & Buki, 2003). Finally, the Quick Discrimination Index measures both cultural diversity and gender equity issues and is particularly useful in assessing racial and gender biases (Ponterotto, Potere, & Johansen, 2002).

Falender and Shafranske (2004, p. 249) listed multicultural competencies required of clinical supervisors, which are reflected in the following questions:

- Do you have a working knowledge of the factors that affect your worldview and the worldview of your supervisees?
- Are you aware of your own cultural self-identity, and are you competent in addressing issues of diversity with supervisees and clients and their families?
- Are you able to perform multimodal assessment of the multicultural competence of trainees, including self-ratings, observational ratings, and supervisor and client ratings?
- Do you model diversity and multicultural competence for your supervisees throughout the supervision process?

- Do you model respect, openness, and curiosity toward all aspects of diversity and explore its impact on behavior, interaction, and therapy and supervision processes?
- Are you able to initiate discussion of diversity factors in supervision?

Clinical supervisors must recognize the potential for cultural bias to play a role in evaluating the performance of supervisees. Supervisors' expectations exert a strong influence on students' performance; when expectations are high, students often rise to the occasion and improve their performance. Similarly, expectations that students will do poorly often result in less-than-optimal performance.

Clouten and colleagues (2006) noted that "when physical therapist students fail to make a smooth transition from the classroom to the clinic, the main problem is seldom lack of knowledge or inadequate psychomotor skills. Difficulties may come from a lack of professional behaviors" (p. 2). They surveyed 192 physical therapy clinical instructors regarding their expectations of and the performance of their minority supervisees. They found that

> Clinical instructors noted a difference in performance between majority and minority students. Results suggest that minority students in general would benefit from further preparation in communication and interpersonal skills and that they are stronger than majority students in stress management and the effective use of time and resources. (p. 11).

The authors emphasized that clinical instructors need to learn to attend to all of the needs students have and to increase their awareness of the challenges that minority students face.

Clinical supervisors should begin dialogues on cultural issues with their supervisees early on in the relationship, but the questions they ask must be timely and not be perceived as threatening. For example, they may ask supervisees if it is okay to discuss issues that may be deeply personal to them. Open-ended questions are particularly useful and will not only give the supervisor insights into the supervisee but also lead supervisees to insights as to how they view the clients they are treating. Haynes, Corey, and Moulton (2003) suggested the following list of questions for fieldwork educators to use in such conversations:

- How do you describe your cultural identity?
- What does it mean to you to identify with this group?
- If you were to think about the multiple layers of culture, which would you identify as the various cultural groups to which you belong?

- In what ways do you think your ethnic identity might affect your role as therapist?
- Are you able to identify, at this time, ways in which our cultural differences or similarities may affect our supervisory relationship?
- How would you self-evaluate yourself in terms in terms of your knowledge and comfort when discussing cultural issues?
- If you find yourself in a cultural discussion that is uncomfortable, can you identify what is it that you find awkward or threatening? Where might you have learned this? Would you be able to tell me that you find this discussion uncomfortable?
- What types of academic training, professional conferences, workshops, or seminars have you attended in the area of multicultural competency?

 Learning Activities

1. Think about your childhood and the cultural lessons you learned growing up. How do these influence your practice of supervision?

2. Reflect on a time in your life when you were in the minority. How did this make you feel? Have you ever experienced bias or prejudice from others? How does this affect your supervisory style?

3. In evaluating your own multicultural awareness, reflect on the following questions (Haynes et al., 2003, p. 141):

- What lens do I view the world through?
- What is my definition of culture?
- What is my cultural heritage?
- What cultural groups do I identify with primarily?
- How did I learn my cultural values?
- What has my experience with other cultures been, and what has my perception of these cultures been?
- How might my beliefs affect my ability to supervise effectively?
- How do I define the relationship between culture and occupational therapy?

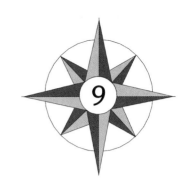

Legal and Ethical Issues in Clinical Supervision

As gatekeepers of the profession, clinical supervisors will continue to be heavily involved with ethical standards for practice. The most instrumental approach to this responsibility is to be well-informed and personally and professionally sanguine. Both are accomplished by continually putting ethics in the foreground of discussion, contemplation, and practice. In this case, perhaps more than any other, supervisors' primary responsibility is to model what they aspire to teach.

(Bernard & Goodyear, 2004, p. 72)

This chapter reviews legal and ethical issues related to clinical supervision in fieldwork and practice and discusses the rights and responsibilities of supervisors and supervisees. As Bernard and Goodyear (2004) pointed out, "Litigiousness has become characteristic of United States society" (p. 49), and news headlines involving ethical issues are steadily on the rise. Consumers of health services are increasingly aware of their legal rights, so supervisors need to have a basic level of legal and ethical knowledge related to their relationships with supervisees and clients whom supervisees treat.

Laws and ethics involve two distinct but interconnected concepts. The codes of ethics of most health and mental health professions comprise very broad statements that may leave a great deal of room for interpretation. Laws are specific statutes enacted by the courts, often in response to an incident in which one or more parties were harmed. Behavior that is unethical often becomes grounds for legal action. As the practice of clinical supervision has become more formalized during the past two decades, specific codes of ethical conduct and legislation designed to protect the consumer have been developed.

Legal Issues

Supervisors have a legal duty to provide oversight to their supervisees as a contractual obligation to the supervisors' employer. If a person were hired to be a supervisor for occupational therapists, occupational therapy assistants, or students, then oversight is contractual, although it is always a professional responsibility. For fieldwork educators, there also is a legal, contractual obligation between the academic institution and the fieldwork site. Going back to the definition of clinical supervision, supervisors and fieldwork educators function as "gatekeepers": Students whose performance meets minimal standards for entry-level competence pass; students whose performance is not safe or ethical, or those who do not meet entry-level competencies, receive a failing grade.

> We first encounter fieldwork as a requirement for becoming an occupational therapist, then revisit it again as a professional responsibility. Serving as a fieldwork educator and sharing with students our affirmation for the profession is a primary way to contribute to the profession. (Cohn & Crist, 1995, p. 105)

The primary legal issues that affect supervision are malpractice; liability; duty to warn, protect, and report; due process; confidentiality; and informed consent. Legal statutes that affect supervision are often within state law; in occupational therapy, supervision standards are defined in state practice acts. Occupational therapy practitioners must be knowledgeable about their own state's practice act, including the provisions on scope of practice and supervision guidelines for students and others.

Malpractice

Malpractice is defined as "harm to another individual due to negligence consisting of the breach of a professional duty or standard of care" (Disney & Stephens, quoted in Bernard & Goodyear, 2004, p. 68). Malpractice thus essentially involves negligence. Four elements must be met for a malpractice claim to succeed (Haynes, Corey, & Moulton, 2003):

1. A fiduciary relationship has been established between the supervisor and supervisee. The fiduciary relationship is based on the premise that the supervisor is working to protect the best interests of the supervisee and his or her clients. This relationship is established when the supervisor agrees to provide supervision.
2. The supervisor has demonstrated behavior that is incompetent or has provided services that in some way have fallen beneath the usual standard of care. Inherent in this principle is a breach of duty; the supervisor has failed either to take certain precautions or to exercise good judgment.
3. The client or supervisee has suffered some degree of harm or injury as a result of the supervisor's incompetent practice. This harm can be physical, psychological, or relational.
4. A causal relationship is established between the injury and the supervisor's actions or lack of actions. Causation must be established that demonstrates that a breach of duty occurred.

Liability

There are two types of liability: vicarious and direct. If a supervisee performs treatment on a client that leads to injury while the supervisee is under the supervisor's guidance, then the supervisor can be subject to vicarious liability. Vicarious liability is based on the concept of *respondeat superior;* the person who assumes authority or control over another can be held liable for any damages the other may cause. A finding of breach of duty is not necessary for the supervisor to be held liable.

Supervisors who are negligent in providing supervision can be subject to direct liability. Haynes and colleagues (2003) listed situations that may result in direct liability:

- Letting supervisees practice outside the scope of practice
- Not providing regularly scheduled supervision
- Failing to provide emergency coverage or to identify emergency procedures to supervisees
- Not providing a supervision contract to supervisees
- Failing to assess supervisees' level of competence
- Failing to assess clients that supervisees are treating
- Insufficiently monitoring supervisees' work with clients
- Failing to provide adequate feedback to supervisees
- Violating professional boundaries in supervision.

Duty to Warn, Protect, and Report

The role of supervisor involves informing supervisees about their duty to report as mandated both by the agency or facility and by law (e.g., suspected child abuse). Many policies related to reporting in mental health practice stem from the *Tarasoff* ruling (*Tarasoff v. Regents of the University of California,* [551 P.2d 334, 131 Cal. Rpter. 141976]). In this case, a psychologist and supervisor were held liable for failing to warn a murder victim that a client had made threats against her. This case has become the foundation of many states' confidentiality laws, which state that a client's right to confidentiality may be waived when there is an imminent threat to the individual or to others. Supervisors must ensure that their supervisees understand both confidentiality policies and policies involving the duty to report.

Due Process

In supervision, due process includes providing supervisees with clearly specified performance expectations, outlining procedures for handling untoward events, reviewing policies for disciplinary action, and explaining supervisees' rights and how they may appeal evaluations. In explaining due process, Haynes and colleagues (2003) noted that supervisees have the right to timely feedback, to be informed of how the process of providing feedback to them will proceed, how they can remediate the situation, what the steps for adverse action will be, and the mechanism for appeal. (p. 33)

Student supervisees are afforded due process rights by virtue of being a student in an academic program; fieldwork is considered to be an extension of the educational program.

Confidentiality

Just as clients have the right to confidentiality, so do supervisees. There are some specific laws that govern student confidentiality. The first is the Family Educational Rights and Privacy Act of 1974 (FERPA; 20 U.S.C. · 1232g; 34 CFR Part 99), which protects student records against being released without the student's written consent. Student records include grades, social security number or student identification number, religion, race, ethnicity, gender, citizenship, nationality, or academic standing. Thus, academic fieldwork coordinators cannot tell fieldwork sites whether a student has failed a previous fieldwork placement, what a student's grades are, or any other information about the student. For this reason, most academic programs have the students complete personal data forms that are sent to fieldwork sites. Even if sharing certain information would be beneficial to the student, it cannot be done without the student's consent.

Supervisors should establish written contracts with their supervisees that address the limits of confidentiality, including whether the supervisor may discuss the supervision with a consultant. Haynes and colleagues (2003) suggested that a good way to model professional behavior for supervisees is to directly address confidentiality issues: "By their own behavior, supervisors have a responsibility to model for supervisees appropriate ways of talking about clients and keeping information protected and used only in the context of supervision" (p. 155).

Informed Consent

There are three separate issues involving informed consent in supervision. The first is informed consent with clients, which is effected when clients are admitted to a particular facility and sign a legal statement giving their consent to procedures. Usually this consent is obtained by the admitting office, but in some smaller practices the therapist may be responsible for obtaining it. If supervisees are responsible for obtaining the client's consent, they must understand how to present the information to clients so that the consent is truly informed.

The second category of informed consent involves supervision. Clients should know when students are treating them, and they also must be aware of any supervision that may occur during their treatment. For example, if supervisees audio- or videotape client sessions for review during supervisory sessions, the client must be informed of such practice.

The third category of informed consent is that between the supervisor and supervisee. Students need to be informed who will be reviewing their work and evaluating their performance. In addition, "supervisors, as such, should be allowed the prerogative of informed consent, that is, they need to be fully aware of the heavy responsibility, accountability, and even culpability involved in [providing] supervision" (Stout, quoted in Bernard & Goodyear, 2004, p. 55).

Ethical Issues

Ethical Concepts Defined in the Code of Ethics

Each licensed profession has its own code of ethics. Occupational therapy practitioners must be familiar with the *Code of Ethics* (American Occupational Therapy Association [AOTA], 2005, Appendixes E and F), which provides the following definitions of ethical concepts as applied to the supervisory relationship:

- *Beneficence* refers to "doing good for others or bringing about good for them" and "the duty to confer benefits to others" (p. 6). In supervision, fulfilling this principle means ensuring that supervisees and the clients they treat receive quality services in accordance with best practice.
- *Nonmalificence* means "not harming or causing harm to be done to oneself or others" and "the duty to ensure that no harm is done" (p. 6). Supervisors are obligated to protect the safety of the clients their supervisees treat.
- *Autonomy* refers to "the right of an individual to self-determination" and "the ability to act independently on one's decisions for their own well-being" (p. 6). Supervisors must collaborate with their supervisees in developing goals for supervision.
- *Confidentiality* means "not disclosing data or information that should be kept private to prevent harm and to abide by policies, regulations, and laws" (p. 6). Supervisors respect supervisees' right to confidentiality.
- *Duty* refers to "actions required of professionals by society or actions that are self-imposed" (p. 6). Supervisors have a duty to achieve and maintain levels of competence as both supervisors and therapists. As echoed throughout this book, supervision is an intervention in its own right; competence as a therapist does not necessarily imply competence as a supervisor. Thus, occupational therapy practitioners have a separate duty to obtain additional training in the practice of supervision.

- *Procedural justice* is one of three types of justice (i.e., compensatory, distributive, and procedural) that refers to "assuring that processes are organized in a fair manner and policies or laws are followed" (p. 6). In the practice of clinical supervision, supervisors must ensure that occupational therapy practitioners comply with all legal statutes and with AOTA policies that define the practice of occupational therapy.
- *Veracity* is simply "a duty to tell the truth; avoid deception" (p. 6). Supervisors need to provide accurate information to and about their supervisees. They also need to represent themselves accurately to supervisees, including their qualifications to supervise.
- *Fidelity* refers to "faithfully fulfilling vows and promises, agreements, and discharging fiduciary responsibilities" (p. 6). Occupational therapy practitioners must treat both clients and colleagues with respect, fairness, discretion, and integrity; the same is true for supervisees and fieldwork students. In supervision, practitioners must adhere to confidentiality laws and must be sufficiently familiar with the AOTA *Code of Ethics* and national and state statutes that they can explain them fully to supervisees.
- Supervisors must be aware of how to report ethical breaches of conduct (see "Procedures for Reporting" on AOTA Web site).

Dual Relationships

Another important ethical concept, dual relationships, is included in the codes of ethics of other licensed professions, such as social work, psychology, counseling, and marriage and family therapists, and I discuss it at length here because it is pertinent to the practice of occupational therapy.

Professionals and supervisors are advised to refrain from engaging in *dual relationships,* which include any relationship other than that of supervisor or therapist. The most egregious violation of this principle is engaging in a sexual relationship with a client or supervisee, for which the AOTA *Code of Ethics* specifies severe consequences. But dual relationships also include anything other than the primary relationship the occupational therapist is contracted to provide. The prohibition on dual relationships stems from the power differential in the supervisory relationship. Providing supervision to a close friend, employer, or relative is considered unethical practice. Participation in social events is problematic; if there is potential for abuse of the power differential, then such events should be avoided. For example, your supervisee asks if you want to catch dinner with him or her after work and then pays for it. Or, you are hosting a party at your home for the occupational therapy department, and alcohol will be served. Both of these examples may seem innocent, but they potentially could lead to problems. In the former example, it is best to ask for separate checks; there will then be no appearance of you being paid. In the latter example, what happens if your supervisee has too much to drink at the party? Are you prepared to take their keys? How will they get home? Asking supervisees to do household chores, babysit children, or type papers—all of these involve the potential for coercion and thus are unethical.

Avoiding dual relationships helps supervisors be vigilant in maintaining firm boundaries with supervisees. Supervisors need to avoid close, personal relationships with supervisees that go beyond professional mentoring relationships. Campbell (2000) articulated questions that supervisors should ask themselves in assessing the potential for dual relationships in a proposed activity:

- What could go wrong in this activity? For example, if you are contemplating asking your supervisee to attend a social event, what are the possible ramifications?
- What is the worst-case scenario that could result from participation in this event?
- Is there anything you can do to avoid potential harm to yourself and your supervisee resulting from the activity?
- Are there any alternatives to the proposed action?

Counseling educators Marijane Fall and John Sutton (2004, pp. 76–77) examined a situation—"let's grab a cup of coffee after work"—with the potential to lead to ethical problems. The request might be initiated by the supervisee, and its intent may be overtly harmless. But the authors cautioned the supervisor about the "slippery slope of dual relationship"; the innocent cup of coffee may lead to an invitation to a movie or other social event, blurring the boundaries in the supervisory relationship. These authors suggested some possible responses to an invitation from a supervisee to discuss research questions over coffee:

- "That's a tough one. On the one hand, I'd love the chance to work with you on these research questions. On the other hand, I feel that our supervision relationship could be affected. So thanks, but I'll just have to work my way through these alone." In this response, the supervisor sets clear boundaries and explains the rationale to the supervisee, thus modeling ethical behavior.
- "I really appreciate the offer, but I have an appointment then." In this response, the supervisor is setting a boundary and says no the supervisee's suggestion using an excuse. Although nothing is inherently wrong with this response, it does not educate the supervisee about boundary setting in supervision.
- "Sure. Maybe we could go out for dinner and that new movie afterwards." This is a danger zone! By taking the supervisee's suggestion a big step further, the supervisor is crossing the boundary into unacceptable practice.
- "Thanks. I really appreciate the offer. I think it would be best if we didn't meet." Again, there is nothing inherently wrong with this

response. The supervisor is setting a clear boundary and saying why, but he or she has failed to explain the rationale behind the decision, missing an important teachable moment.

- "Could we spend some time discussing the boundaries of our supervision relationship first so that we both are clear?" With this response, the supervisor is being proactive by ignoring the question and tackling the bigger issue directly. This response not only models appropriate professional behavior but also opens a dialogue that will be educational for the supervisee.

Avoiding Ethical and Legal Misconduct

Supervisors can do the following things to ensure that they do not engage in practices that result in ethical violations or legal transgressions:

- Obtain malpractice insurance. Even when working at a facility that provides malpractice insurance, get your own liability insurance. In the occupational therapy profession, such insurance is relatively inexpensive. Settlements in lawsuits often are beyond the limits of liability insurance provided by employers, and it is sometimes difficult to get a copy of your agency's malpractice insurance policy. The limits of liability from these group insurance policies may not be adequate; some gaps in coverage that may occur, such as financial limits on coverage for occupational therapists or occupational therapy assistants; no provision to pay for lost wages, licensing board hearing reimbursement, and defense costs; coverage for on-site claims only, so any kind of pro bono or volunteer work is left uncovered; and coverage limited to the practitioner's length of employment. By obtaining your own insurance, you will have your own policy in writing so that you know the parameters of your potential liability.
- Be familiar with the *Enforcement Procedures, Occupational Therapy Code of Ethics* (AOTA, 2005a), your state's Practice Act, and the AOTA *Standards of Practice for Occupational Therapy* (AOTA, 2005b), just to name a few. Education is the best prevention.
- Avoid any and all dual relationships.
- Obtain consultation or supervision for yourself when confronted with a difficult supervisory issue.
- Use a written contract for supervision.
- Document all supervisory contacts. Keep a supervision log with the date and time of each and every supervisory contact, along with a brief summary of what was discussed.
- Obtain training in the area of supervision through conferences or workshops, independent reading, and/or courses in supervision.

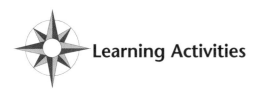 **Learning Activities**

Read through each of the following scenarios,* which were created by Alexander Lopez, JD, OTR/L, Clinical Assistant Professor and Academic Fieldwork Coordinator I for the Occupational Therapy Program at Stony Brook University. Respond to the questions at the end of each scenario.

1. Outpatient Physical Disability Setting (Specialty): Level II Fieldwork (8 Weeks)

In the fourth week of Cara's hand therapy rotation, Cara's performance to date was less than mediocre. In fact, her supervisor, Cailey, was considering giving her a failing grade for her midterm evaluation. Unknown to Cailey, Cara had struggled through her previous Level II fieldwork and only just passed her Level I physical dysfunction fieldwork. She submitted all of her assignments after the due date, and her progress notes contained numerous grammatical and spelling errors. Cara failed to demonstrate an ability to think critically and used the same textbook intervention strategies for many of her clients. Cara had a great work ethic and personality, however, and her clients loved her.

Cara had learning disabilities (attention deficit disorder, dyslexia, and dysgraphia) that impaired her ability to perform certain tasks. Although her secondary school teachers and school psychologists had identified Cara's problems, Cara did not reveal her disabilities to the occupational therapy program. At midterm, Cailey informed Cara that she was failing. Cara then informed Cailey that she had learning disabilities and could improve if reasonable accommodations were made.

- What should Cailey have done when orienting and supervising Cara during the first 4 weeks of fieldwork?
- If Cailey chose to fail her, what would she have to do to ensure that Cara's constitutional rights were not violated?
- After their midterm meeting, what should Cailey do next?
- Are reasonable accommodations required in this situation?
- If reasonable accommodations are made, would Cara be required to provide proof of disability?
- Can Cailey obtain information from Cara's high school?

Source: Case studies reprinted with permission of Alexander Lopez, JD, OTR/L.

2. *Acute Rehabilitation Setting: Level II Fieldwork (12 Weeks)*

Patrick, who had completed 4 weeks of his second Level II fieldwork, had an unhealthy combination of athletic build and know-it-all attitude. Patrick demonstrated poor transfer techniques with his clients. Moreover, he refused to ask for assistance when needed. Patrick tended to perform the same transfers with all of his clients. He squatted, pivoted, and flung the client. Jillian, Patrick's supervisor, provided several instructional sessions on transfer techniques with patients with orthopedic and neurological impairments. Patrick continued to perform transfers with too much thrust.

One day, Jillian observed Patrick in the occupational therapy department performing his characteristic transfer. She rolled her eyes, stated "He is so dense," and returned to her paperwork. Jillian recognized Patrick's poor performance and potential to do harm, yet she did nothing more to correct him. Two weeks later, Patrick was sent to a client's room to assist the physical therapist in getting the client out of bed. Patrick arrived before the physical therapist and decided to perform the transfer without assistance. The client was a 70-year-old morbidly obese man who had recently had a total hip replacement. During his attempt to transfer the client, Patrick dropped the client. As a result of the fall, the client sustained a dislocation of his affected leg.

- Identify the potential issues.
- What do you think is meant by "Patrick has an unhealthy combination of athletic build and know-it-all attitude."?
- What should Jillian have done after observing Patrick transfer clients improperly? Is she liable of any wrong doing? Why or why not?
- What do you think should have occurred when Patrick dropped the client?

3. *Inpatient Mental Health Setting: Level II Fieldwork (12 Weeks)*

Brenda was in the 6th week of her mental health fieldwork rotation. Brenda had a history of mental illness; she had disclosed her disability to the academic institution but not to the fieldwork site. She took prescription medication that allowed her to function effectively. However, because of the stress associated with fieldwork, she decompensated. Brenda was absent on five occasions, of which three were excused. Brenda reported to work late on five other occasions. Brenda had great rapport-building skills and was a dynamic group facilitator.

One Friday, she left the door open to a cabinet for storing scissors and other sharp devices in the recreation room. Three hours later, a staff occupational therapy assistant, Alex, found the cabinet door open and locked it. Alex informed Brenda's supervisor about the cabinet door; the supervisor had observed Brenda leaving the cabinet door open on one other occasion. Alex also informed the supervisor of another incident that occurred during her first week, when Alex observed Brenda leaving the door open on leaving the unit. A client attempted to leave the unit, and Alex intervened. Alex told Brenda about the incident and warned her to be more careful when working.

- Identify the problem areas.
- At midterm evaluation, how would you rate Brenda's performance to date?
- What other feedback would you provide at her midterm evaluation?

4. *Pediatric Therapy: Level II Fieldwork (12 Weeks)*

By the 8th week of Jackie's fieldwork experience, her performance was fair to good. According to the site's fieldwork manual, Jackie should have been seeing 8 clients a day, but Jackie was currently seeing 6 clients per day. Jackie was very intelligent and had an outstanding academic record. She had excellent writing skills and a firm understanding of occupational therapy theory. Jackie had poor interpersonal skills, however. When given critical feedback, she made tactless facial gestures. She sighed when spoken to and was often argumentative. Although she demonstrated good client–therapist interaction, she had not been well received by the other staff, who described her as arrogant and unpleasant.

- Identify the problem areas.
- How would you rate Jackie's performance?
- What would you do on her final evaluation?

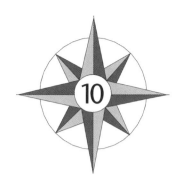

Feedback in Clinical Supervision

Because of its value, some people have called feedback the breakfast of champions. But it isn't the breakfast, it's the lunch. Vision is the breakfast. Self-correction is the dinner. Without vision, we have no context for feedback.

(Covey, 1994, p. 247)

This chapter covers one of the most significant tools for influencing learning that a supervisor has: feedback. I will describe what feedback is, what makes it effective, and what contributes to defensive responses from supervisees. As Westberg and Jason (1993) stated, "Feedback is central to many aspects of our lives" (p. 297).

What Is Feedback?

Students and practitioners often use *feedback* synonymously with *constructive criticism,* but a better definition of feedback is "information given to indicate the level of competence that has been achieved in performance of a task. Feedback therefore can be positive or negative depending on whether the task was completed well or not" (Rose & Best, 2005, p. 63). Hoffman, Hill, Holmes, and Freitas (2005) defined feedback as "information that supervisors communicate to their supervisees about aspects of their skills, attitudes, behavior, and appearance that may influence their performance with clients or affect the supervisory relationship" (p. 3).

Feedback is a crucial motivating factor in learning. In 1912, Edward Thorndike, a psychologist, performed one of the first experiments on feedback (cited in Westberg & Jason, 1993, p. 297). He divided participants into three groups and asked each group to draw lines of different lengths. The first group did not receive any feedback on their performance. The second group was given partial feedback; they were told whether the lines were too long or too short but not the degree of error. The third group was given specific feedback on their performance, including exactly how far off their lines were from the assigned lengths. The first group's performance did not improve over time, and the second group showed slow improvement, but the third group was able to learn to draw the exact length assigned in only a few trials. These results showed that people learn best from feedback that is both timely and specific.

Bernard and Goodyear (2004) found that when supervisees were asked to reflect on the supervision they received, they described the type and adequacy of the feedback. Other researchers found similar results; Lehrman-Waterman and Ladany (2001) linked satisfaction with supervision to the quality and time-liness of feedback, and Magnuson, Wilcoxon and Norem (2000) found that when supervisees did not receive enough feedback, they qualified the supervision they received as "lousy."

Numerous studies in the health education literature (e.g., Scheidt et al., 1986; Stillman, Sabers, & Redfield, 1976) have reported that when compared with students who receive no feedback, students who receive feedback perform significantly better in clinical practice. Irby (1986) reported that students gave the lowest satisfaction scores in clinical education to receiving feedback and direction. Studies comparing supervisee perceptions to supervisor perceptions of feedback frequently have found that supervisors felt they were giving adequate feedback, but students did not share that perception. For example, in a study by Collins, Cassie, and Daggett (1978), 79% of physicians felt that they were giving adequate feedback to residents during medical rounds, but only 49% of the residents felt they had received feedback on their performance. A case study report by Friedlander, Sigel, and Brenock (1989) found that few feedback comments were made in supervision.

In a more recent study by Ladany and Melincoff (1999), 98% of supervisors of graduate student counselors admitted to withholding some feedback from their supervisees. This begs the two-part question, Why do supervisors withhold feedback, and under what conditions do they find it more difficult? Hoffman and colleagues (2005) examined all of the different conditions under which supervisors find it difficult to give feedback, particularly negative feedback. The factors they identified included fear of negative consequences from giving a subordinate negative performance feedback; embarrassment about giving negative feedback, especially if the supervisee had been promoted; and the desire to avoid confrontation with the supervisee. The authors' overall finding was that supervisors were reluctant to provide negative feedback because of concerns about its relevance and the desire to avoid a negative reaction from the supervisee. Supervisors found it easier to give feedback about clinical performance issues than about factors that related to the supervisory relationship, personality issues, or professional behavior. In addition, they found it easier to give both positive and negative feedback when the supervisee was receptive and open to receiving feedback and when factors such as a strong supervisory relationship, good timing, and outside support were present.

Why Is Feedback So Important?

Westberg and Jason (1993) identified a number of reasons for supervisors to find ways to increase the amount of feedback they give to supervisees. Among these reasons are the following:

- Effective feedback facilitates learning. Without feedback, learning is delayed and can be incomplete.

- Supervisees value feedback. That being said, some supervisees value it more than others. Some supervisees ask for it, and some even ask for it to excess, which also can be problematic. But the emphasis has to be on constructive feedback—in other words, feedback that supports learning.
- Timely feedback is essential to enable students to succeed. It is particularly distressing to academic fieldwork coordinators when they get a call from a fieldwork educator in the 10th week that a student is going to fail. The coordinator rushes out to the site, and the student reports that he or she did not know about the impending failure until that day. This type of feedback is too little, too late. Likewise, the day of the final fieldwork evaluation or annual performance review is not the time to provide feedback for the first time.
- Students need adequate feedback to correct their mistakes and avoid bad habits. Supervisors must prevent as many mistakes as possible and ensure that any that are made are corrected immediately, particularly if these mistakes will cause harm to the client. In some situations, however, the supervisor can permit the supervisee to make a mistake and then learn from the mistake, so as not to repeat it again. Again, this is only possible if the mistake is benign and will not cause harm to the client or supervisee. Showing supervisees the correct way to do something through role modeling is a good way to start, but supervisors also must take the time to observe them doing it correctly.
- Feedback encourages positive behavior. If supervisors want supervisees to adopt certain behaviors, they have to catch them doing those behaviors right. Effective teachers help others recognize their strengths and their growing edges. But in the early stages of learning, behavior must be reinforced to become stronger.
- Feedback ensures that supervisees make accurate assumptions. Although a great deal of learning consists of trial and error, supervisors need to explain the reasons behind what they do to encourage supervisees' clinical reasoning skills and reflective practice. For example, supervisees who do not receive feedback may assume that they are failing because they have not received any feedback that they are in fact doing well. If supervisors look unhappy while observing their supervisees, the supervisees might assume that their supervisors are unhappy because of their level of performance rather than distressed for some unrelated reason. Timing of feedback is an art. In some situations, the supervisor can interrupt the supervisee to provide him or her with feedback; however, to do so in front of a client may cause more harm than good. It undermines the supervisee's confidence, as well as the client's trust in supervisee. Also, some feedback is better

received privately than in front of the supervisee's peers, which may cause embarrassment and undermine confidence.

- Regular feedback decreases anxiety on tests and final evaluations. If supervisors give regular feedback, supervisees feel more confident because they know how they are doing. In fact, confidence is built much more effectively by regular feedback than by a grade on a test.

Types of Feedback

Rose and Best (2005) pointed out that effective feedback has two functions: It gives supervisees information about their actual performance, and it motivates them to perform better. A supervisee's receptivity to feedback depends on a number of factors, including the task, the setting, the supervisee's learning style, and the type of feedback used. The authors listed eight types of feedback and their advantages and disadvantages:

1. Written feedback gives supervisees visual, permanent feedback, allowing them to compare their progress over time. The disadvantage is that it is time consuming, and often supervisees see only the negative feedback. Written feedback also does not allow for discussion or collaboration between supervisor and supervisee.

2. Verbal feedback is a more active type that generally leads to and facilitates discussion. The down side is that it can be time consuming, and supervisors may find it difficult to give face-to-face feedback that is negative.

3. Audiovisual feedback is given after supervisees perform the intervention, allowing them to concentrate on the client. Supervisors and supervisees review the recording together. Supervisees may experience increased anxiety levels with this feedback type if they are uncomfortable being recorded or cannot tolerate watching or listening to themselves. Videotaping is better than audiotaping, which does not record nonverbal behaviors, in providing supervisees with an accurate view of the treatment session. The client's consent must be obtained to record the treatment session, which may alter the tone of the session.

4. Most supervisees prefer receiving individual feedback in privacy, where no one else can hear about their mistakes. One-on-one feedback allows supervisors to address more sensitive issues, but it is time consuming and may be one of the reasons supervisors are switching to group feedback.

5. For the time-pressed practitioners, group feedback represents maximum efficiency. However, supervisees who are not comfortable in group situations may be silent throughout sessions, requiring supervisors to elicit their input directly. Both supervisees and supervisors find it difficult to share and discuss negative feedback in groups unless the supervisors actively promote this discussion through techniques such as self-disclosure and role modeling. For this purpose, a group consists of more than one supervisee. It is used frequently with students on fieldwork, particularly if the fieldwork educator uses a collaborative learning model. Group supervision actually is a more effective supervision technique than individual supervision, because it uses group dynamics and feedback from peers. Bernard and Goodyear (2004) provided a formal definition of group supervision:

> Group supervision is the regular meeting of a group of supervisees
>
> - With a designated supervisor or supervisors,
> - To monitor the quality of their work, and to
> - Further their understanding of themselves, as clinicians, of the clients with whom they work, and of service delivery in general.
>
> These supervisees are aided in achieving these goals by their supervisor(s) and by their feedback from and interactions with each other. (p. 235)

6. Direct feedback involves the provision of specific feedback—for example, "We're here today to discuss the evaluation you performed with Mrs. Smith; you followed the outline we use here and performed all the components without error." Direct feedback is supervisor driven, which means that it does not always allow supervisees the opportunity to problem solve and self-reflect about the efficacy of their performance. Supervisees should be encouraged to listen for direct feedback from clients to reduce their overreliance on feedback from the supervisor.

7. Indirect feedback involves drawing conclusions about one's own performance from the outcome. For example, a supervisee conducting a problem-solving group with psychiatric inpatients can self-assess his or her performance on the basis of how well the group went, the behaviors the clients demonstrated, and

the extent to which the group objectives were met. This type of feedback comes from reflective practice and may be difficult at first for fieldwork students; however, it is an intended learning outcome and should be encouraged.

8. Peer feedback comes from fellow students or colleagues and is frequently a part of collaborative learning. The supervisor must set explicit expectations for the tone of such feedback and encourage regular provision of peer supervision.

Improving the Effectiveness of Feedback

To be effective, feedback needs to be accurate, timely, specific, objective, useful, and desired by the supervisee. Rose and Best (2005) listed many characteristics of effective feedback. The following paragraphs discuss some of these characteristics.

Feedback is most effective when it is obtained from multiple sources. In providing feedback to supervisees about their professional behavior, supervisors should not comment solely on their attire, for example, but also on their verbal communication and written documentation. Supervisors can communicate observations that also have been made by other members of the treatment team to add credibility to the feedback.

The source of the feedback must be credible in the eyes of the supervisee. Supervisees will discount feedback that comes from someone whom they do not consider competent, a good role model, or knowledgeable in the particular practice setting. In addition, supervisees will be unlikely to accept feedback that they have done something incorrectly if it is something they have seen their supervisors do. Effective supervisors do not say, "Do as I say, not as I do."

Feedback that is effective takes into account the supervisee's stage of professional development. Feedback on entry-level skills is more appropriate for new supervisees than feedback on advanced practice skills. Similarly, timing is important; supervisees are more ready for feedback at some times than at others. For example, if a student just finished providing an intervention and it did not go particularly well, the student may be visibly upset, perceiving this as a failure. I usually allow time for the supervisee to regain his or her composure before providing feedback. If I give the feedback while the student is emotional, the effectiveness of the feedback will be lost. I might suggest that the student take a break and that we'll discuss it when he or she returns. Students typically rate their own performance, particularly in the beginning of fieldwork, as abysmal. They may need more support and encouragement early on to counteract their own negative views of themselves. When I provide feedback, I do not say "Let's discuss the good and bad points of what you did"; rather, I do say "Let's discuss what went well and what are your 'growing edges'." *Growing edges* implies where additional learning needs to occur.

If the supervisee has never before performed a particular task, then the feedback should reflect that this is a new or emerging skill. All feedback should acknowledge any discrepancy between the specific task and the just-right challenge.

Effective feedback uses different methods. Supervisors should match the feedback to the supervisees' learning style. For those who are visual learners, written feedback may be more beneficial. For those who are more kinesthetic, opportunities should be provided to demonstrate skills and receive immediate feedback. Sometimes the best format for feedback depends on the task. For example, with documentation skills, I find that written feedback works best, but with transfer skills, demonstration works best.

Feedback needs to be clearly understood and based on the facts. The information supervisors give to supervisees should be objective and free from bias. Feedback should not give the impression, for example, that the supervisor does not like the particular student or supervisee or the school that he or she came from. In addition, supervisors need to confirm that supervisees accurately hear what they have intended to communicate. Asking supervisees to summarize the feedback given to them is a good way to check their comprehension; if their recounting contains inaccuracies, then the supervisor can correct them. Supervisors can say "Tell me what you heard me saying to you about your performance" or "Can you summarize for me what we just discussed?"

Feedback that is effective relates to specific behavior or data. Supervisors must be specific and give examples. Saying "your performance leaves much to be desired" is too vague. What parts or aspects of the performance need to change? Supervisors need to back up their feedback with specific examples rather than generalizations about their performance.

Effective feedback focuses on the behavior, not on the person. Supervisors' task is to evaluate performance. Whether they like the supervisee is irrelevant. The supervisory role does not include changing supervisees, only shaping their behavior. Supervisees who are very sensitive may perceive feedback as an attack on their personality. In such cases, it is important for the supervisor to reiterate what he or she said about the behavior and to emphasize that he or she is not talking about the supervisee's failure as a person. Readers who have had the experience of failing a student on fieldwork understand the importance of explaining this distinction: The student's performance is failing, not the student as an individual, and the effective supervisor tries very hard to make sure that this message gets heard.

Words that describe rather than evaluate result in more effective feedback. Many people are defensive when it comes to hearing feedback about their behavior. Focusing on the skill-building aspect of the feedback, rather than on the underlying cause of why supervisees did what they did, can minimize defensiveness. For example, if a supervisee is frequently late for work, focusing on strategies to get to work on time may result in less defensiveness that asking the person why he or she is always late.

Effective feedback occurs close to the actual event. The success of the "One-Minute . . ." book series (Blanchard & Johnson, 1981; Blanchard & Zagarmi, 1985) is based on the principle that to increase motivation, people need to be acknowledged for doing something right at the time they are doing it. When supervisors give feedback days or weeks after the event, it is not as helpful as discussing the event immediately afterward.

Honoring the person's privacy increases the effectiveness of feedback. Giving negative feedback when others are around to witness it results in shame and humiliation for the supervisee. Supervisors should be sure to give feedback, particularly of a more sensitive nature, in an area where others cannot see or hear the conversation.

Feedback should be built into the daily routine. If feedback is woven into the everyday fabric of the worksite, supervisees will view it more as a continuous process rather than a single event. Ongoing feedback helps supervisees stay on track and avoid feeling dread when the supervisor says "Come into my office ." The just-right challenge applies to this aspect of feedback: Feedback should be frequent enough so that supervisees know how they are doing but not so frequent as to prevent opportunities to self-reflect and independently problem solve.

Supervisees should be encouraged to ask for feedback. Feedback is more effective when supervisees ask for it of their own volition. Feedback is more to likely to motivate the supervisee to change performance when he or she solicits it voluntarily.

Supervisees' receptivity to feedback is influenced by their level of self-esteem. The lower the supervisee's level of self-esteem, the more he or she will rely on feedback from external sources. The lower the supervisee's self-esteem, however, the more likely he or she is to focus on the negative aspects of the feedback. Those with higher self-esteem focus more equally on negative and positive feedback.

"Sandwiching" positive and negative feedback increases its effectiveness. When giving a supervisee negative feedback, the supervisor can start with positive feedback and then give the negative feedback, ending with more positive feedback. In this way, the supervisee is more likely to avoid focusing on the negatives.

Feedback must be relevant to the individual. In addition to being timely, feedback needs to relate explicitly to something the supervisee said or did. Supervisors should make every effort to ensure that the feedback addresses the supervisee's interests; supervisees do not need to become like their supervisors to be successful.

Supervisees may need time to formulate a response. Supervisors need to wait for supervisees to digest, process, and respond to feedback. Supervisors may need to be silent for a moment or even say to the supervisee, "Think about this before you respond." When the feedback is negative, supervisors need to be prepared for a defensive, angry, or even tearful response. They should ask supervisees how they see the situation or even how they might have given someone else this feedback if they were in the supervisor's shoes.

Feedback should be related to the goals outlined in the learning contract. Supervisees are more likely to be receptive to feedback when the supervisor relates it to the goals of the learning. For example, a supervisor might say, "One of the things you said you wanted to work on was setting limits with clients, so I'm going to give you some feedback that will help you achieve that goal." If negative feedback is given, supervisors should help supervisees establish a goal that addresses how they will learn to do something differently.

Feedback using the first person is most effective. Beginning in the first person establishes a dialogue and makes the recipient of the feedback less defensive—for example, "I like the way you made eye contact with the client before asking her a question." Statements beginning with "You" put the recipient on the defensive.

A question format eases the delivery of negative feedback. Using questions to elicit discussion can help make negative feedback sound less negative—for example, "Can you describe the frame of reference you're using?" Supervisors should be careful when they use questions, however, especially those that start with "Why did you" because they can invite a defensive response.

Negative feedback should be delivered in carefully chosen language. Negative feedback is especially difficult to hear when delivered in language that is derogatory or inflammatory. Supervisors must always avoid statements like "You're never going to make it here unless you toughen up" or "You're going to fail fieldwork if you don't start working harder." Nonverbal communication and tone of voice also should be considered when delivering negative feedback; supervisors should avoid folding their arms across their chest in an angry posture, looking at their watch, or using an angry tone of voice.

Physicians Felise Milan, Sharon Parish, and Michael Reichgott (2006) provided a model for providing effective feedback called the PEARLS mnemonic as a way for supervisors to remember the critical elements in providing feedback and provide a supportive environment for supervisees. The letters in the mnemonic stand for the following words:

P = partnership for joint problem–solving,
E = empathic understanding,
A = apology for barriers to learner's success,
R = respect for learner's values and choices,
L = legitimation of feelings and intentions, and
S = support for efforts at correction. (p. 43)

The authors suggested using the stages-of-change model (Prochaska, DiClemente, & Norcross, 1992), which includes *precontemplation, contemplation, preparation, action,* and *maintenance,* to assess how ready supervisees are to change a particular behavior:

- *Stage 1—Precontemplation.* Clients in this first stage have not yet admitted that they have a problem; consequently, they use denial and other defenses to use as a justification for their problem.
- *Stage 2—Contemplation.* Clients just have begun to admit they have a problem. Their acknowledgment permits attempts to increase their awareness and knowledge related to the problem.
- *Stage 3—Preparation.* Clients are now starting to figure out how they will go about "fixing" their problem; they have developed an awareness of the benefits of change, which have outweighed any barriers to change. Activities include considering all of the various options they have to eradicate the problem, develop a strong commitment to the change process, and write out a detailed plan for changing their behavior.
- *Stage 4—Action.* Clients have initiated the behaviors they need to effect the change they planned. People in their lives will be able to observe these behaviors as evidence that the client is trying to make a change. This stage requires at least 6 months, at which point clients may be ready to move to the fifth stage.
- *Stage 5—Maintenance.* Clients maintain the changes they made, although they must be vigilant to any risk factors that may lead to a relapse to the unwanted behaviors. Clinicians should spend a great deal of time helping the person identify the warning signs, as well as helping them to develop coping strategies for relapse. Once the changed behavior has become totally integrated so that it has become so automatic that no possibility exists of reverting to a former behavior, then the goal of termination has been achieved.

During the feedback process, the educator can "diagnose" the learner's stage of readiness and employ focused interventions to encourage desired changes. The educator can help the learner to identify discrepancies between current behavior and stated goals, as well as barriers to change. (Milan et al., 2006, pp. 43–44)

I end this chapter where I began, by quoting the work of Steven Covey (1994, p. 247):

But with a clear sense of vision, we can use feedback to help us achieve a greater integrity. We have the humility to recognize that we have blind spots, that getting other perspectives will help us improve the quality of our own. We also have the wisdom to realize that feedback tells us as much about the people from which we receive it as it does about ourselves. The responses of others reflect not only how they see us, but also how well they feel we do those things that are important to them. Because people are important to us, and because part of our leadership is creating shared importance, this dimension of feedback is vitally important as well.

Learning Activities

1. Answer each of the following questions* as honestly as you can (from Westberg & Jason, 1993):

- Am I able to establish and maintain a climate of trust in which supervisees welcome feedback from me?
- Do I tell supervisees that I will be giving them regular feedback? If so, do I tell them when and how they will be receiving this feedback?
- Do I give supervisees feedback in an environment that is conducive to receiving feedback?
- Do I give feedback to supervisees in a timely manner?
- Do I keep in mind the supervisee's learning style and goals for learning when I provide feedback?
- Do I encourage supervisees to give themselves feedback on their performance?
- Do I support my feedback with specific examples from the supervisee's actual practice?
- Do I deliver feedback without bias or judgmental language?
- Do I provide feedback in a supportive manner?
- Do I provide the right amount of feedback that a particular supervisee can handle?
- Am I comfortable giving supervisees negative feedback? Can I help them turn it into a learning lesson?
- Do I encourage supervisees to ask for feedback? Do I also encourage them to tell me when the feedback is difficult to hear?

*Source: Adapted from *Collaborative Clinical Education: The Foundation of Effective Health Care,* by Jane Westberg and Hilliard Jason, © 1993. Reproduced with the permission of Springer Publishing Company, LLC, New York, NY 10036.

- Do I acknowledge that not all supervisees will respond the same way to feedback?
- Do I focus my feedback on specific behavior of the supervisee, rather than making judgments about him or her as a person?

If you have difficulty with any of these statements, use that feedback to create a learning plan for yourself, or discuss the items with a trusted colleague or mentor.

2. How do you feel when you are given constructive feedback? Have you ever taken this feedback as a criticism of you as a person? Describe that situation.

3. How do you feel about giving feedback to others? Can you think of a time you gave feedback well? Describe the situation. Can you remember a situation in which you either did not give feedback when you should have or did not give it effectively? Describe the situation.

4. Think of a time when you received negative feedback from a supervisor. How did this make you feel? What could the supervisor have done to deliver the feedback more effectively?

5. "Try to recall a feedback experience that was particularly powerful for you as a learner in the practice setting. Describe the incident. Identify your own thoughts and feelings related to the feedback. How was the feedback delivered? Consider the language of the feedback. How did this impact on you as the learner? Analyze the incident and consider why it was so critical to your learning. Identify elements of good practice and areas of development related to the delivery and content of the feedback. How does your own approach to giving feedback to learners match up to your ideal?" (Cross et al., 2006, p. 116)

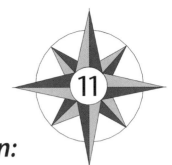

The Process of Clinical Supervision: Tools of the Trade

Good teaching cannot be reduced to technique; good teaching comes from the identity and integrity of the teacher. Good teachers possess a capacity for connectedness. They are able to weave a complex web of connections among themselves, their subjects, and their students so that students can learn to weave a world for themselves.

(Palmer, 1998, pp. 10–11)

This chapter covers some significant resources that clinical supervisors need to have in their supervision toolbox—learning contracts, supervision contracts, supervision logs, and supervision formats. Some of these tools have particular formats, whereas others are more knowledge based. I discuss the knowledge, skills, and techniques involved in using these tools of the trade.

Learning Contracts

Learning contracts (sometimes called *negotiated learning agreements*) are used widely in clinical education in many professions. Some clinical educators use learning contracts only when a supervisee requires remediation. This limitation is unfortunate, because a learning contract also can be an invaluable tool for students having no difficulty in learning. Brookfield (1987) identified learning contracts as a primary means to enhance self-direction, because they provide both a format that gives the learner control over what he or she learns and the evaluative criteria to assess learning. Knowles (1980) described learning contracts as central to adult education principles; they provide a method and means for expressing the learner's needs and interests (see also Knowles, Holton, & Swanson, 2005). Furthermore,

> learning contracts provide a vehicle for making the planning of learning experiences a mutual undertaking between a learner and his or her helper, mentor, teacher, and often, peers. By participating in the process of diagnosing his or her needs, formulating personal objectives, identifying resources, choosing strategies, and evaluating accomplishments, the learner develops a sense of ownership of and commitment to the plan. (Knowles et al., 2005, p. 266)

In field-based learning, the learning objectives may not be clear initially to the student, and learning contracts make the learning objectives explicit (Knowles, 1980). Matheson (2003) observed that learning contracts are an effective way to link theory and practice, helping students transfer skills and knowledge from the classroom into the clinical practice setting.

Some disadvantages to using learning contracts have been identified, including the amount of time it takes to create them (Whitcombe, 2001), lack of understanding on the part of fieldwork educators (Matheson, 2003), and anxiety and frustration for students if they are not prepared to develop learning contracts (Cross, 1996). In addition, the fieldwork site needs to have a culture that supports self-directed learning (Rose & Best, 2005). Whitcombe (2001) suggested that the success of the learning contract depends on the fieldwork educator's attitude. Kennedy-Jones (2004) described the following characteristics of an environment that is supportive of learning contracts:

- Practitioners can communicate thoughts, feelings, knowledge, and experience in an atmosphere of safety.
- Trust is present so that learners are allowed to learn from their own experience and make their own decisions.
- Educators relinquish some of the control typical of more traditional learning settings so that learners can select their own learning methods.
- Educators are aware of the types of communication that support self-directed learning, as opposed to language that inhibits such learning.
- Educators facilitate student learning by giving advice and feedback when needed and support students' independent learning.

Some students have a great deal of anxiety about formulating their own learning contracts; such students typically have had no prior exposure to active learning and are accustomed to being passive recipients of knowledge. They will need the supervisor's support and encouragement to develop learning objectives that focus on what they want to learn rather than what they think the supervisor feels they need to learn.

Rose and Best (2005, p. 253) identified the following steps in developing a learning contract and provided some guiding questions for learners:

- Assess the learner's prior experiences and learning: "Where have I been?"
- Identify the learner's current level of knowledge and skills: "Where am I now?"
- Develop learning goals and objectives: "Where do I want to go next?"
- Create a proposed plan of study that will meet goals and objectives: "How will I get there?"

- List the resources that will be needed to meet learning goals: "What will I need to help me?"
- Identify evaluative criteria for assessing the extent to which the learning goals were achieved: "How will I know that I have reached my goals?"

Knowles and colleagues (2005, pp. 266–271) identified a slightly different, six-step process for learners to use in developing a learning contract:

1. Diagnose your learning needs by identifying the gap between where you are right now and where you want to be in a particular skill or aspect of knowledge.
2. State the learning objectives, with an emphasis on what you want to learn rather than what you want to do. Objectives can be in the areas of learning a skill, acquiring knowledge, or personal or professional growth.
3. Specify the learning resources and strategies that you need to accomplish your goals. Resources can be human or material, and strategies are techniques and tools.
4. Describe the types of evidence you will collect to demonstrate that you have accomplished the learning objectives.
5. Specify how the evidence will be validated by describing the criteria you will use to evaluate the types of evidence you listed in Step 4. For example, if you identified an examination as the type of evidence for demonstrating that learning objectives have been met, then a passing grade would be how you validate the evidence. If the learning objective is a particular skill and the evidence is demonstrating the skill to the supervisor, then the validation would be satisfactory performance in demonstrating the skill.
6. Review the learning contract with friends, colleagues, and the supervisor to elicit their reactions and suggestions. You might ask them about the following:

   - Are the learning objectives clear and realistic?
   - Can they identify additional learning objectives for you?
   - Are the resources and strategies appropriate to the objectives?
   - Might there be other resources and strategies you could use?
   - Is the type of evidence relevant to the learning objectives? Would this evidence convince them?
   - Can they suggest other types of evidence you could use?
   - Do the evaluative criteria make sense, and are they also convincing?

- Can they identify any other ways you could validate the evidence?
7. Carry out the learning contract you developed.
8. Evaluate the learning that you have achieved.

Kember and colleagues (2001) suggested that it is not the learning contract itself that is helpful to the learning process but rather the communication and collaboration that occur between the student and clinical educator. Thus, learning contracts not only benefit the student but also foster professional development in the supervisor. See Figure 11.1 for a sample learning contract.

Supervision Contracts

A supervision contract is broader than a learning contract and extends to specifying the structure of the supervision in addition to what is to be learned. Although it is not a legal contract, it is a written agreement that spells out the mutual responsibilities of both the supervisor and the supervisee. Such contracts promote due process by ensuring that both parties know what is expected of the other. Falender and Shafranske (2004, p. 209) identified the following key components of a supervision contract:

- Goals and objectives mutually agreed on by supervisor and supervisee
- Methods for measuring the supervisee's progress
- Time frames for goal attainment
- Developmental needs and strengths of the supervisee
- Competencies of the supervisor
- Activities both parties agree to do
- Supervision procedures
- Amount of, frequency of, and time to be spent on supervision
- Location and modality of the supervision provided
- Opportunities to be provided within the practice setting
- Evaluation process to be used with the supervisee.

The supervision contract also promotes informed consent, empowering the supervisee to collaborate with the supervisor on what will be accomplished in supervision.

In advocating for the use of supervision contracts to occupational therapy supervisees, Early (2000) emphasized that

> supervision is a two-way undertaking, and you as supervisee must understand that you contribute to the process. As a supervisee, you are responsible for your own learning. Your supervisor's role is to facilitate your learning, not to teach you step-by-step. Thus, the supervisee is expected to identify and attempt to solve problems

SAMPLE LEARNING CONTRACT

Name: Donna M. Costa, MS, OTR/L

Position: Student in doctoral program at University of Indianapolis

Learning Objectives

I expect to be able to learn

1. To be able to submit articles for publication to *OT Practice,*
2. To be able to conduct program evaluation studies, and
3. To be able to construct a graduate-level course in fieldwork supervision.

Learning Resources and Strategies (with target dates in parentheses)

Strategy 1
a. Obtain guidelines for authors from *OT Practice* (5/06).
b. Write first draft of co-authored article on trip to Ukraine and submit it to mentor and coauthor at University of Indianapolis for feedback and correction (7/06).
c. Submit article to *OT Practice* for editor's review (8/06).

Strategy 2
a. Take doctoral-level course in program evaluation at the University of Indianapolis (10/06).
b. Complete all pre-course and post-course assignments to obtain corrective feedback (10/06).
c. Design and administer program evaluation instrument to students at Stony Brook University, then analyze results and write paper (11/06).
d. Submit report to professor at University of Indianapolis for grade and corrective feedback (12/06).

Strategy 3
a. Research and read existing literature on existing training courses in clinical supervision (12/06).
b. Design graduate course syllabus for entry-level students at Stony Brook University, conduct course, and obtain student feedback (2/07).
c. Construct a post-professional graduate course syllabus and submit to mentor at University of Indianapolis for corrective feedback (4/07).

Evidence of Learning Objective Being Achieved

1. Publication of article in *OT Practice.*
2. Successful completion of program evaluation.
3. Submission of course syllabus on clinical supervision for fieldwork educators.

Evaluation of Learning and New Learning Objectives (consistent with lifelong learning)

FIGURE 11.1. Sample learning contract.

resourcefully and to make independent use of opportunities
afforded by the library, the Internet, professional organizations
and events, and clinical opportunities such as in-services. (p. 506)

A supervision contract may seem like a formality, but it is a practical tool that
can prevent misunderstandings later. Figure 11.2 provides a sample contract;
actual contracts must be tailored to fit the needs of the supervisee, the supervisor, and the practice setting.

Supervision Logs

It is essential that supervisors maintain written documentation of all supervisory sessions with supervisees. This record-keeping does not have to be elaborate
and add much to the busy practitioner's workload. For instance, I just keep a
sheet in the supervisee's folder, which has a space for the date and time of supervision and brief notations on significant issues or discussed cases. If the supervisee later says, "You didn't provide me with enough supervision," I can
produce a list of the dates and times I did provide the sessions. Also, the sheet
can be completed during supervision sessions, which models the importance of
documentation for the supervisee.

Documentation is important for liability purposes, because it provides a
record of what was discussed in supervisory sessions. In the event that a client
or supervisee takes legal action, the supervisor will be able to produce a time-
line of supervisory sessions, cases discussed, and supervisee progress. If a supervisee's competence is questioned, the log will document the nature of the
problems discussed, the supervisor's response, and any corrective action taken.
Supervision logs further provide a record of the number of supervisory hours
the supervisor provided, as well as documenting the supervisor's skills.

At a minimum, supervision logs should contain the following:

- Date of session
- Time and length of session
- Location of supervision (e.g., office, clinic)
- Supervision modality (e.g., one on one, group, video)
- Cases reviewed
- Treatment plans
- Review of therapeutic activities and modalities used
- Concerns shared with supervisee
- Suggestions or recommendations given to supervisee.

The length of the log is not as important as its thoroughness in recording the
objective facts of the supervisory sessions. The log should contain facts, behavioral observations, quotes, and other pertinent data and should leave out the
supervisor's subjective feelings about the supervisee.

The parties listed below will work together during the supervisee's 12-week Level II fieldwork experience, which begins on _____ and ends on _____.

Supervisee's name:	Supervisor's name:
_____	_____
1. I agree to meet with my supervisor at least once each week, or more often if necessary, to discuss issues, concerns, and questions.	1. I agree to meet with my supervisee at least once a week, or more often if necessary, at the agreed-on times.
2. I will follow through with my assigned responsibilities, which include compiling occupational profiles, performing evaluations, submitting weekly progress notes, following group protocol, leading one group daily, presenting a case study to the treatment team, and presenting an in-service to the department staff.	2. I will suggest resources that the student can use to perform his or her assigned tasks, and I will provide learning activities to enhance learning.
3. In addition, I will develop a learning contract to give to my supervisor that identifies the learning goals I wish to focus on during this fieldwork experience.	3. I will notify the student in advance of any changes in assignments or times of supervision sessions.
4. I agree to abide by the facility's rules, maintain confidentiality guidelines, respect the rights of others, and abide by AOTA's *Occupational Therapy Code of Ethics* at all times.	4. I will collaborate with student to identify learning goals and provide direction and resources to ensure that learning goals for the fieldwork assignment are met.
	5. I will review all documentation that the student gives to me and provide written feedback within one week.
	6. I will provide the student with a midterm evaluation on or about _____ and a final evaluation on _____.

Date: _____   Supervisor: _____

Supervisee: _____   Facility: _____

Note. Adapted with permission from Figure 24.1 in Early, M. (2000). *Mental health concepts and techniques for the occupational therapy assistant* (3rd ed., p. 507). Philadelphia: Lippincott.

FIGURE 11.2. Sample supervision contract.

The supervisor should encourage the supervisee also to keep a log of the supervisory sessions; taking notes helps supervisees focus on using supervision effectively and understanding the supervisor's recommendations or suggestions. Documenting supervisory sessions is a good habit that will prepare supervisees to begin supervising their own students.

Two formats for supervisee logs are the reflective journal and the summative log. Reflective journal writing is an excellent tool to help supervisees go deeper into the learning experience. One way to help supervisees structure a reflective journal is to ask them to describe each day or week how they felt about what happened in addition to recording simply what happened. (Further detail on journal writing is provided in Chapter 12.) Summative logs can provide fieldwork students with structure for their learning. Students are asked to write down weekly what happened, what they learned, what learning goals were met, and what they want to focus on the next week. The log can serve as an ongoing record of what supervisees learned each week and help them prepare for supervisory sessions.

Supervision Formats

In the original model of occupational therapy (and other professional) fieldwork education, one professional took one student and taught the student all that he or she knew. This is now referred to as the one-on-one model. Over time, alternative models of supervision have developed out of the need to train more students and to reflect different learning theories. Some research has examined the outcomes of different supervision formats, but more is needed. Although many supervisors are comfortable with supervising only one student, other formats have advantages, particularly in taking into account individual learning styles. Which format the supervisor uses depends on a number of factors, including time constraints, the organizational structure of the facility, management style, personality factors, and the supervisor's comfort zone. These formats are summarized in the paragraphs that follow.

Individual or one-on-one supervision is the most frequently used format. Supervisees recount their work to their supervisors, and the supervisors make suggestions, ask questions to promote reflection and clinical reasoning, and plan for future supervision sessions. This format provides supervisors with the most control over supervisees' learning and makes it easy for supervisors to monitor supervisees' performance when providing line-of-sight supervision. The relationship between supervisor and supervisee is a critical component of this format. The limitations of this format include an overreliance on self-report by supervisees, limitations on opportunities to engage in collaborative learning, and the risk of supervisees becoming dependent on their supervisors for feedback (Martin et al., 2004, Steele-Smith & Armstrong, 2001).

Group or one-on-two (or more) supervision is based on the collaborative learning model, in which one supervisor provides supervision to a group of supervisees. Like the one-on-one model, this format relies on self-report by supervisees; however, it adds the element of group dynamics and encourages collaborative learning. The relationship with the supervisor becomes less authoritative as supervisees learn to accept feedback from each other in addition to the supervisor. The role of the supervisor is to guide and facilitate questioning and clinical reasoning skills. Students frequently become more self-reliant and independent when this format is used as they learn how to use resources other than their supervisor.

In group supervision, more time is required of supervisors for planning, and they should familiarize themselves with the principles of collaborative learning. Supervisees also should be provided with articles about or descriptions of collaborative learning so that they understand the expectations. Supervisors need to be comfortable in a group format and with group dynamics. Supervisees, particularly students, may become competitive, and this tendency must be managed so that it is a constructive force and not a destructive one. Students who are reticent or quiet will have difficulty with this format, and supervisors must draw them out gradually in a way that supports their learning. Lastly, sensitive situations need to be addressed individually, and evaluations should always be done in a one-on-one session.

Two-on-one supervision provides the supervisee with two supervisors; this format often is helpful in settings where supervisors are part-time employees or share caseloads. It can be an excellent way to mentor new supervisors by allowing them to participate in providing supervision without having all of the responsibility. Some serious limitations, however, can occur in this format, particularly when the two supervisors rarely see or speak to each other (e.g., because they work on different days or in different locations) or when they do not share the same philosophy of treatment or supervision. In such cases, the supervisee may be caught between conflicting sources of information and expectations. It needs to be made clear up front how supervisors will communicate with each other and with the supervisee, and strategies for increasing communication between the two supervisors may be necessary.

Sometimes two-on-one supervision involves supervisors from different disciplines; this format often is used in role-emerging practice, like in a community mental health practice where an occupational therapy practitioner and a social worker share supervision, as well as settings where the supervisor is available for a limited number of hours a week and someone else needs to be available to the supervisee. The primary supervisor is typically from the supervisee's discipline, and a professional from a different discipline is designated as the supervisor when the primary supervisor is not available. This format can enrich the supervisory experience by providing the student with another viewpoint, but care must be taken that the supervisors do not present conflicting information. Supervisors from disciplines other than occupational therapy need to understand occupational therapy's scope of practice and must defer to the occupational therapy supervisor in discussing aspects of care they are not familiar with. Because students sometimes feel that they are being shortchanged when the occupational therapy supervisor is unavailable, occupational therapy supervisors need to explain as part of the orientation why this format is being used and suggest ways students can use it to their advantage in meeting their learning goals.

Audio- or videotaped supervision minimizes reliance on the supervisee's self-report, permitting the supervisor to see or hear what actually transpired in the treatment sessions. The supervisor can see or hear nuances in the supervisee's responses that might be missed in the one-on-one format. This format, however, is not without disadvantages. An additional consent must be obtained from the client that specifies who will view or listen to the tape and what will happen to the tape afterward (e.g., Will it be destroyed or retained? If retained, for how long, and where?). In addition, some people are anxious or self-conscious while being recorded, and this factor needs to be taken into account when listening to or viewing the tape. Bernard and Goodyear (2004) and Campbell (2006) provide some excellent suggestions on how to use videotaping as a supervisory method or technique. While videotaping, unlike audiotaping, allows the supervisee to view their own performance and self-reflect, it does create even more anxiety for the supervisee. The supervisor will have to be attentive to this and help the supervisee focus on what is important in the session. Some suggested strategies follow, based on Campbell (2006):

- Decide on the purpose for videotaping and identify this to the supervisee. For example, a supervisee brings the same problem repeatedly into supervision, such as "I'm having trouble starting sessions with clients," and verbal problem-solving has not been helpful. Suggest that recording a session (if the client approves) might be a way for both of you to better understand the difficulty in starting sessions.
- Pay attention to confidentiality. Tapes need to be treated the same way as client's medical records and should be kept in a locked location. Avoid placing identifying information on the outside of the tape. View the tape in a private setting, not at home or work where others may see it.
- Prepare the supervisee for viewing tape by selecting the section or sections to be discussed in supervision.
- Reduce supervision anxiety. I don't know anyone who is ecstatic over seeing his or her image on videotape. Be vigilant to the supervisee's anxiety level throughout the supervision session. Have the supervisee

identify something he or she thinks he or she did really well in the session and view that first.

- Emphasize the training aspect of viewing the tape (i.e., the specific learning goals). Ask the supervisee to tell you how he or she thinks this will help him or her.
- Either the supervisor or the supervisee can stop the tape at periodic intervals to discuss what happened. Regardless of who stopped the tape, allow the supervisee to comment first to minimize the power differential. This technique needs to be done frequently; at least one author has suggested that the attention span for watching one's own videotape is only about 4 minutes (Whiffen, 1982).
- Be aware of the number of critical responses given to the supervisee to minimize anxiety in the supervisee. Keep reiterating the goals of the learning activity.
- Be aware of and address the resistance the supervisee may be exhibiting. Put yourself in his or her shoes.
- End with restating the goal of the learning activity and ask the supervisee to summarize what he or she learned in terms of the original goals.

Co-treatment or live supervision is an *in vivo* supervision format in which the supervisor and supervisee work together in the treatment session. The supervisor's role can be passive if the purpose is simply to provide line-of-sight supervision or more active if the supervisor is co-treating with the supervisee. This format enables the supervisor to use role modeling and facilitate active learning by demonstrating skills to the supervisee rather than just describing them. Although this format may be optimal for the supervisee, it may overwhelm the client and also may undermine the client's trust in the supervisee if the supervisor is presented as the expert. It also can reduce supervisees' self-confidence, particularly if they feel that the supervisor has knowledge and skills that they do not yet possess.

E-mail or remote supervision is a by-product of the information age and is frequently used in role-emerging practice settings or in rural areas. For supervisors and supervisees who are comfortable with technology-facilitated communication, it can be an excellent vehicle for providing supervision. It can be time consuming for both parties, however, and subtleties of interpersonal communication such as affective responses and nonverbal communication often are lost in e-mail communication.

Team supervision is used most often in large hospitals or health care facilities. While group supervision most typically involves several supervisees from the same discipline, such as a group of Level I fieldwork students or therapists in a large occupational therapy department, team supervision uses work units of supervisees, who are likely to be from different disciplines, such as an acute psychiatric unit (where the psychiatrist conducts weekly team supervision) or a burn unit (where the unit director discusses cases weekly with the members of the treatment team). In this format, one professional typically supervises everyone on a work team or unit. The supervisor sometimes teaches via demonstration; for example, a psychiatrist or psychologist may interview a client in front of the treatment team (or behind a two-way mirror) as a teaching tool for interviewing techniques or diagnostic formulation. Role-playing and prerecorded videotaped demonstrations also are used in team supervision.

In peer supervision, which usually augments one-on-one supervision, peers provide feedback to each other without the presence of the supervisor. This format can be an excellent vehicle to support self-directed learning and increased problem-solving skills and clinical reasoning in participants. It works well when all parties value the peer supervision equally and when no one person dominates the sessions. For students, peer supervision can increase the amount of supervision received when a supervisor can spend only limited time with supervisees. Peer supervision also is a good method for occupational therapists to continue their professional development once they have left school by getting together with colleagues periodically to review cases and share treatment strategies. Campbell (2006) noted, however, that peer supervision is not effective when there is a great disparity among colleagues in terms of education or amount of clinical experience. It also does not work well when the work environment is undergoing internal changes and tensions are running high. When trust among peers is not at an optimal level, supervisees may not feel safe disclosing information to each other.

 Learning Activities

1. To explore using videotaping as a method for supervision, make a few practice tapes for yourself before you use this format with supervisees. Make a videotape of a treatment session (be sure to have the client's written consent first) and then view it privately, noting your own reactions to being recorded. This experience will help you understand your supervisees' reactions to this supervision format. Watch the video a second time, but this time, create a checklist of things you want to focus on learning, and watch the video as if you were your own supervisor. Ask yourself the following questions:

- What happened in the session?
- What did you do well?
- How did you respond to the client?

- What might you have done differently?
- Were there any issues involving cultural diversity in the session?
- Did you become aware of something in watching the video that you were not aware of during the session?
- How did the client respond to being videotaped?
- What was effective in promoting desired intervention process and outcomes?

You also might try letting a trusted colleague view the tape and provide you with feedback. Again, note your reactions to hearing feedback based on the videotape.

2. Think back to the supervisors you have had. What formats of supervision did they use? What worked well? What didn't work well, and why?

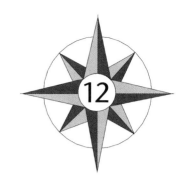

Reflective Practice and Collaborative Learning

Supervisors can only take others to a depth of exploration and reflection that they have personally and professionally experienced themselves.

(Long & Chambers, 1996, p. 51)

In his seminal book *Educating the Reflective Practitioner,* Schön (1987) wrote the following:

> In the varied topography of professional practice, there is a high, hard ground overlooking a swamp. On the high ground, manageable problems lend themselves to solution through the application of research-based theory and technique. In the swampy lowland, messy, confusing problems defy technical solution. The irony of this situation is that the problems of the high ground tend to be relatively unimportant to individuals or society at large, however great their technical interest may be, while in the swamp lie the problems of greatest human concern. The practitioner must choose. Shall he remain on the high ground where he can solve relatively unimportant problems according to prevailing standards of rigor, or shall he descend to the swamp of important problems and nonrigorous inquiry? (p. 3)

This chapter takes readers into the "swampy lowland," focusing on the process of reflective thinking that takes the practice of clinical supervision to a deeper level. Developing reflective thinking skills and practice is the path to becoming a reflective practitioner and a means of facilitating one's own professional growth. This process also can be used in the supervisory process as a way to increase critical thinking and reflective practice in students and supervisees. This chapter also includes material on collaborative learning, a related process for taking learning to a deeper level.

What Is Reflective Practice?

Schön (1987) is credited with advancing knowledge of reflection and the ways it can be used to enhance learning. Educational reformer John Dewey (1933), however, was the first to define it: "Reflective thinking is the active, persistent and careful consideration of any belief or supposed form of knowledge in the light of the grounds that support it and the further conclusion to which it tends" (p. 9). According to Dewey, students cannot be taught exclusively what they need to know, nor does experience alone itself lead to learning. The student

> has to see on his own behalf and in his own way the relations
> between means and methods employed and results achieved.
> Nobody else can see for him, and he can't see just by being "told,"
> although the right kind of telling may guide his seeing and thus
> help him see what he needs to see. (p. 151)

Experiential learning must be accompanied by the type of thought process that Dewey (1933) named *reflective thinking*. In addition, Dewey said, this reflective thinking must be accompanied by three attitudes or characteristics—open-mindedness, whole-heartedness, and responsibility.

Fish and Twinn (1997) expanded on Dewey's concepts, identifying the following characteristics of reflective practitioners (see also Rose & Best, 2005):

- Are open to new ideas and ways of doing things
- Are interested in improving the quality of their work for their patients' benefit
- Are passionate and enthusiastic about their work
- Identify their work as meaningful and worthwhile
- Are able to admit their limitations and current level of competence
- Act in a morally and ethically responsible manner
- Recognize the importance of their values and beliefs in providing patient care
- Practice holistically using a problem-solving approach
- Look for collaborative solutions to workplace issues and concerns
- Engage in critical conversations about their practice and with their inner selves, thus leading to new knowledge and insight about their practice.

This list of attributes suggests the importance of practitioners being open to discovery and curious about exploring elements of their practice in such a way that problems are viewed as challenges and as opportunities to learn to do things differently.

Reflective Practice

Dewey (1933; see also Rose & Best, 2005) identified five phases in the reflective process of examining a problem in practice. When practitioners encounter a problem in their practice, they should refrain from doing the first thing that pops into their head. Rather, they should take the time to explore the process in five phases:

- *Phase 1* is characterized by ideas being converted into suggestions that then lead to further inquiry.
- *Phase 2* is a problem-solving stage in which the problem is examined in the context of the bigger picture.
- In *Phase 3,* the process of intellectualization is used to explore the problem and develop insights and suggestions that lead to a working hypothesis, which the practitioner can begin to test.
- *Phase 4* is the reasoning phase, in which practitioners expand their thoughts about the problem and consider alternatives.
- In *Phase 5,* the alternative solution or strategy is tested and the outcomes—positive and negative—contribute to learning.

This process illustrates what reflective practitioners go through when encountering a problem in their practice. As Wales, Nardi, and Stager (1993) stated, practitioners "delay action long enough to understand the situation as fully as possible, to consider the end that they hope to achieve, to generate and weigh up as many options as they can and to plan before they take action" (p. 182).

Thus, reflection is a way that practitioners can deepen their practice and further their professional growth, and certain situations should trigger reflective thinking. Brown and Ryan (2000) identified some of these triggers:

- Something that went really well,
- A crisis,
- A situation that made the practitioner uncomfortable,
- A situation in which something that usually worked well did not work, or
- An occasion when a usual explanation was not sufficient, leading to the need to discover a new explanation.

Another vehicle for deepening reflective practice is to examine *critical incidents,* or incidents or situations that were unexpected in some way. Perhaps the results of an intervention were a surprise or of concern or led to confusion. Examples of critical incidents are

- An action that made a significant difference to the outcome in therapy,
- An action or event that exceeded the practitioner's expectations,
- Something that did not go as well as planned,
- An event or situation that challenged the accepted way of doing things,
- An event that affirmed or exemplified a theory or practice the practitioner learned in school, and
- Something that illustrated the need to integrate theory and practice.

Fish, Twinn, and Purr (1991) described another method for facilitating written reflection, which they named *strands of reflection*. The four strands of reflection are the factual strand, the retrospective strand, the substratum strand, and the connective strand. These four strands and the relevant reflective questions are described in the paragraphs that follow (see also Brown & Ryan, 2000).

The *factual strand* involves reflecting on procedural knowledge and examining the situation using a narrative of the events and processes. The narrative is written in the first person, as if the person was still in the situation. This type of reflection also is known as *debriefing*. The components of the factual strand include

- *Recalling the practical situation:* Who was there? Where did the situation take place? Why did the situation occur?
- *Telling the story in chronological order:* What was the planned course of action? What actually happened? How was what happened different from what was planned? Can you pinpoint the critical incidents? What questions arose in your mind? Which of these questions offer you opportunities for learning? What do you think you need to learn more about? How did you feel and react at the time? What have you learned from this?
- *Identifying ideas for future practice:* What should happen next in your practice? What could happen, considering your responses to these questions?

The *retrospective strand* focuses on thinking about an event or incident in a reflective manner, drawing from practice and developing sensitivity and imagination by increasing one's appreciation of the wider perspectives of practice. Questions to ask in the retrospective strand are as follows:

- Looking back at the event, what patterns of behavior and/or responses can you see?
- What did you expect to get out of the event?
- What were the overall goals and intentions? Were these goals and intentions achieved?
- What viewpoints on the event might other practitioners have to offer? In other words, how might they have felt about the situation?
- How does the context you identified in the factual strand relate to what actually happened?
- What existing knowledge did you draw from?
- What new things did you learn?
- How can you describe the interactions that occurred between the people involved in the situation? What do you make of these human relationships as a whole?

- Thinking back on the language used in the situation, what might it tell you?
- What new discoveries did you make as a result of the event?
- What reasons, motives, and emotions might have contributed to the actions in this situation?
- What were the connections between the critical incidents?

The *substratum strand* involves exploring and discovering the underlying beliefs, assumptions, and value judgments about the events and ideas described in the factual strand and retrospective strand. In the substratum strand, the practitioner is encouraged to recognize that there may be no one right answer and to tolerate divergent perspectives. The following questions are helpful in the substratum strand:

- What customs, traditions, and rituals were brought to the situation or were apparent?
- What beliefs, dogmas, prejudices, or emotions were brought to the situation or were apparent?
- Where did these elements come from? What is their origin?
- What basic beliefs and assumptions underlay the actions, emotions, and decisions identified in the factual and retrospective strands?
- What beliefs about your existing knowledge and your newly gained knowledge emerge as you reflect? How did you gain that knowledge, and how will you use it?
- What do you think about the theory and practice implicit in the situation? What do you think about the way you are reflecting about the situation and your new learning?
- How might you explain the kinds of evaluation and justification that you have used to guide this reflective process?
- Which theories did you base your actions on?
- What can you say about the outcomes of your actions? Were the anticipated outcomes yours or someone else's?
- How would you describe your relationship with your work?

In the *connective strand,* the practitioner integrates his or her new understanding of the situation and expanded knowledge base from the three previous strands. This strand involves examination not only of the practitioner's own views, experiences, and reflections, but also of those of colleagues and other professionals with whom the practitioner works. Some questions that promote thinking at this level include

- What have you learned from this entire situation?
- How does it relate to your prior experience?
- How might it relate to future experiences?

- What do you now understand about what motivated your own practice?
- How do your own thinking and actions mesh with the wider context of your practice?
- How might you modify your thinking and actions in a similar situation in light of this experience, your thoughts about it, further reading, and reflection?
- What implications does your reflective thinking have for future practice?

Professional Artistry

Schön (1987) coined the term *professional artistry* to refer to

> the kinds of competence practitioners sometimes display in unique, uncertain, and conflicted situations of practice. Note, however, that their artistry is a high-powered, esoteric variant of the more familiar sorts of competence all of us exhibit every day in countless acts of recognition, judgment, and skillful perform-ance. What is striking about both kinds of competence is that they do not depend on our being able to describe what we know how to do or even to entertain in conscious thought the knowledge our actions reveal. (p. 22)

Titchen and Higgs (2001) offered another definition of *professional artistry* as a "uniquely individual view of practice within a shared tradition involving a blend of practitioner qualities, practice skills, and creative imagination process-es" (p. 275). Professional artistry is present when practitioners make a commit-ment to providing high-quality practice. According to Fish and Twinn (1997), such practitioners' work

> encompasses not the pre-specified list of individual competencies that take no account of context, but a repertoire of skills, abilities, capacities, professional knowledge, personal attributes, personality and ability to work with other professionals, together with . . . flexibility, educational understanding, moral awareness and professional judgment. (p. 154).

Brown and Ryan (2000) used the image of an iceberg to illustrate the com-plexity of clinical reasoning in professional practice (Brown & Ryan, 2000). Only one-ninth of the iceberg is visible above the water, and only "actions" are above the water line—that is, visible to others. "Experience" hovers at the water line, because some of practitioners' experience is visible to others—that is, what they tell others about themselves or list in a resume or curriculum vitae. The other components of clinical reasoning—knowledge, feelings, expectations, assumptions, attitudes, beliefs, and values—are hidden beneath the surface of the water: They are visible only deep inside each practitioner.

Schön (1983) described several types of reflective thinking that practitioners can use to enhance their professional practice. One of these is what he named *reflection-in-action,* which occurs when practitioners face a problem that forces them to stop, think, and engage in problem-solving on the spot. Practitioners often refer to this as "thinking on one's feet." Schön described it well:

> The practitioner allows himself to experience surprise, puzzlement, or confusion in a situation which he finds uncertain or unique. He reflects on the phenomenon before him, and on the prior under-standings which have been implicit in his behavior. He carries out an experiment which serves to generate both a new understanding of the phenomenon and a change in the situation. (p. 68)

When encouraging reflection-in-action with a supervisee in teaching them something new, supervisors frequently use demonstration to facilitate learning. Schön described three ways to use demonstration:

1. *Follow me* is best used in the early stages of learning. The supervisor demonstrates a treatment or technique in its entirety while the supervisee watches, making notes of what he or she observes. Next, the practitioner repeats the demonstration but this time stops at certain key points to emphasize their importance, to explain what he or she is doing, and/or to emphasize to the learner the reasoning behind what he or she is doing. Lastly, the practitioner repeats the entire treatment or technique in its entirety again, this time without stopping, so that the supervisee can observe with his or her new insight or knowledge.

2. *Joint experimentation* is useful for practitioners who want to teach or learn an advanced skill or knowledge. The supervisor initially takes the lead but then stops at some point and asks the supervisee how to proceed or what comes next. The practitioner then proceeds using the supervisee's suggestion, stopping periodically to explain or discuss the validity of what the supervisee suggested. Thus, the supervisee learns by increasing his or her clinical reasoning skills in a series of supported steps.

3. *Hall of mirrors* is an active learning method in which either the supervisor or the supervisee performs a skill, pausing at key moments to engage in a reflective discussion. The supervisee is asked to think about his or her feelings and to identify any

153

challenges he or she might be experiencing in carrying out this skill. Both the supervisor and the client provide feedback to the supervisee.

Schön (1987) wrote that reflection-in-action involves a three-stage process (see also Rose & Best, 2005, p. 149):

- *Stage 1:* The practitioner allows himself or herself to "experience surprise, puzzlement, or confusion" when confronted with a situation in which he or she feels unsure or uncertain about how to act or proceed.
- *Stage 2:* The practitioner begins thinking about the situation, bringing to the surface his or her thoughts and understanding of the situation. The practitioner analyzes the situation further to restructure how he or she thinks and feels about the situation.
- *Stage 3:* The practitioner can now engage in an "on-the-spot experiment" that will lead to a new way of looking at or understanding the situation.

In addition to reflection-in-action, Schön (1983) also developed a concept he called "reflection-on-action," which refers to the thinking process that practitioners engage in after the situation is over. Reflection-on-action can happen through writing (as in a journal) or discussing the situation in supervision or with a colleague. The practitioner explores why he or she acted as he or she did and attempts to view the situation from different perspectives. Schön elaborated as follows:

> When a practitioner makes sense of a situation he perceives to be unique, he sees it as something already present in his repertoire. . . . It is, rather, to see the unfamiliar, unique situation as both similar to and different from the familiar one, without at first being able to say similar or different with respect to what. The familiar situation functions as a precedent, or a metaphor, or . . . an exemplar for the unfamiliar one. (p. 138).

Reflective Journaling

Reflective journaling can be a powerful medium for enhancing reflective thinking in practitioners and in their supervisees. It is a form of writing for the purpose of learning. Holly (1997) defined *journaling* as follows:

> Not merely a flow of impressions, it records impressions set in a context of descriptions of circumstances, others, the self, motives, thoughts, and feelings. Taken further, it can be used as a tool for

analysis and introspection. It is a chronicle of events as they happen, a dialogue with the facts (objective) and interpretations (subjective), and perhaps most important, it provides a basis for developing an awareness of the difference between facts and interpretations. (p. 5)

This type of writing, however, must be structured in such a way to elicit reflective thinking. Simply asking supervisees to write about what happened will not lead them to the kind of deep learning involved in reflective practice. Boud (2001) suggested the following headings or prompts for journal writing:

- *Return to the experience:* What happened? In this step one mentally revisits what happened.
- *Attend to your feelings:* How did you feel? Whether the emotions surrounding the event or experience were positive or negative, one needs to examine and feel them to learn from them.
- *Re-evaluate the experience:* How did it happen? What does it make you think about? In this step, one connects old information and prior experiences with current experience, leading to new learning.

Thus, the practitioner works through a process in the reflective journal entries that enables him or her to extract meaning from events and experiences that have occurred. Boud (2001) also described using journal writing with three kinds of reflection, which he conceptualized as (a) reflection in anticipation of events, (b) reflection in the midst of action, and (c) reflection after events.

Blake (2005) identified many learning goals that can be achieved through reflective journals, including

- Discovering meaning,
- Making connections between what one learned in the classroom and one's own life experiences,
- Instilling the values of the profession,
- Recognizing the perceptions of others,
- Reflecting on one's professional role,
- Improving one's narrative writing skills,
- Developing critical thinking skills,
- Increasing problem-solving skills,
- Processing affective experiences, and
- Taking care of oneself.

When a supervisor assigns journaling to supervisees, the supervisor may grade journal entries or simply write comments. It is important to tell the supervisee in the beginning who will be reading the journal entries and, if they will be graded, what the scoring rubric will be. For example, I routinely give Level II fieldwork students daily reflective journal assignments. I let them know that I am the only one who will be reading them and that I will write my comments on the entries themselves. I let them know that these assignments help me understand their learning process. I instruct them to write not about what happened, but about how they felt about what happened. As I read their journal entries, I write questions in the margins aimed at getting students to think deeper the next time they write a journal entry. Journals are well worth the time invested, particularly when the supervisor is not full-time at the site. Reading journal entries gives the supervisor insight to developing critical thinking and clinical reasoning skills, as well as any affective processes. As faculty members, grading student papers is not usually a favorite part of the job, but it is an important one. Similarly on fieldwork, as fieldwork *educators,* it is a learning activity requirement that goes with the territory. How can we assess student learning if we do not grade student journal entries?

Several articles have suggested ways to grade students' journal entries. In their study examining the validity of grading reflective journal entries, Williams, Sundelin, Foster-Sargeant, and Norman (2000) gave students and educators the following five criteria and then examined the differences in their responses. These criteria could serve as guideline to give fieldwork students:

1. Supervisees should describe the learning event or situation, as well as prior knowledge, feelings, and attitudes and current knowledge, feelings, and attitudes. This description answers the question, What happened?
2. Supervisees should analyze or re-evaluate the learning event, issue, or situation in relation to their prior knowledge, feelings, and attitudes. This analysis answers the question, What is your reaction to the learning event, issue, or situation?
3. Supervisees should verify or confirm that the learning event, issue, or situation changed their prior knowledge, feelings, or attitudes. This confirmation answers the question, What is the value of the learning event, issue, or situation that has occurred?
4. Supervisees should reflect on their responses to the first three questions to gain a new understanding of the learning event, issue, or situation. This reflection answers the question, What is your understanding of the learning event, issue, or situation?
5. Supervisees indicate how they think the learning event, issue, or situation might affect their future behavior. This reflection generally leads them to clarify an issue, develop a skill, or resolve a problem or conflict and answers the question, How will you approach the same or similar events, issues, or situations in the future?

Journal entries that are purely descriptive and that focus on what happened rather than analyzing the learning event, issue, or situation are given the minimum grade. Journal entries that are nonreflective serve no learning purpose and must be discouraged. I tell my students, "I don't want to know what you did, but I want to know how you felt about what you did." Students who are writing just to fulfill the assignment need to be told it is not acceptable, because superficial entries never will accomplish the goal of reflective practice.

A group of physical therapy educators (Plack, Driscoll, Blissett, McKenna, & Plack, 2005) integrated concepts developed by Schön (1983, 1987), adult education professor David Boud (2001; Boud, Keogh, & Walker, 1985), and educational theorist Jack Mezirow (1991) to create a grading rubric for journal entries. Their students attended a lecture on reflective practice before beginning their field placement. Journal entries were graded for the presence of four types of element, which the authors defined for the purposes of this study (Plack et al., 2005, pp. 206–207): (1) time-dependent elements, (2) content-dependent elements, (3) stage-dependent elements, and (4) levels of reflection.

Time-dependent elements include the following:

- *Reflection in action* occurs while in the midst of an activity and is the result of an on-the-spot decision.
- *Reflection on action* occurs after the action has been completed; the student describes an event and attempts to better understand the situation, his or her actions, or the outcomes.
- *Reflection for action* occurs in anticipation of a situation, when the student begins to plan for the future to improve either the situation or the outcome.

Content-dependent elements include the following:

- *Content:* The student explores the problem or experience from a number of different perspectives (going beyond description) to understand it better.
- *Process:* The student describes the strategies or processes involved in problem-solving or managing a situation and may begin to explore other strategies.
- *Premise:* The student recognizes and explores his or her own assumptions, values, beliefs, and biases and may begin to seek multiple perspectives and alternative explanations.

Stage-dependent elements include the following:

- *Returns to experience:* The student describes the experience and the aspects of it he or she considers significant.
- *Attends to feelings:* The student acknowledges and begins to work with feelings that resulted from the experience.

- *Re-evaluates:* The student reappraises the situation in light of past experiences. The student might associate the experience with past experiences in order to link a new concept to previously learned knowledge; begin to integrate new information; attempt to validate his or her new insights, thoughts, and perceptions; and integrate this new meaning into his or her way of being.

Levels of reflection include the following:

- *Nonreflection:* No evidence of reflection is present; the supervisee describes experiences but without analyzing or questioning them.
- *Reflection:* Evidence of reflection is present; the supervisee has paused to reflect on what happened in order to explore and better understand the experience.
- *Critical reflection:* There is evidence that the student has engaged in critical reflection and has stopped to explore the problem, its source, or the assumptions underlying the problem. The student revisits the experience, critiquing his or her assumptions and thought processes, demonstrating evidence of recognizing assumptions, and perhaps beginning to modify biases or assumptions.

McAllister (2000) suggested three stages of reflection to facilitate the kind of deep learning that is the goal of journaling. Clinical supervisors can create prompt questions for each stage to help their supervisees write truly reflective journal entries:

- *Stage 1:* Return to the experience.
- *Stage 2:* Pay attention to the emotions.
- *Stage 3:* Re-evaluate the experience through the processes of association, integration, validation, and appropriation.

Reflective journaling can be a powerful learning process, but some supervisees resist it, because it can be uncomfortable at times. As Holly (1997) noted,

> Habit, motivation, and sometimes our own biases and unrecognized needs move us to behave in ways that are uncomfortable when we question ourselves. We allow ourselves to be vulnerable when we question ourselves. Our humanness shows. We sometimes feel threatened by change and the discomfort that accompanies the cognitive dissonance arising from the difference between our image of ourselves and our behavior. (p. 14)

To summarize, supervisors need to remember that supervisees must understand why they are being asked to reflect over and over and how they can use the tools and methods listed in this chapter to deepen their professional practice. Westberg and Jason (1991) identified the following as reasons why reflective practice is a valuable professional development activity:

- It helps practitioners both identify and build on existing knowledge.
- It enables practitioners to identify where they have deficits or gaps in knowledge.
- It helps practitioners identify errors or mistakes they make in the decision-making process.
- It is helps practitioners generalize information from one situation to another similar one that may occur in the future.
- It helps practitioners integrate new knowledge with existing knowledge.
- It forces practitioners to examine their biases and assumptions that they may be unaware of but that may affect patient care.
- It helps practitioners become more aware of the feelings and emotions they experience.
- It helps practitioners become empowered after gaining ownership of new insights that emerge from their reflective thinking.
- It helps the supervisees increase their competencies and skills.
- It reinforces the importance of lifelong learning and of developing early the good habit of continually engaging in learning activities and processes.

Collaborative Learning

Collaborative learning is both a process and a method for supervising students (as well as for continuing one's own professional development), particularly when working on interdisciplinary teams or seeking to enhance team development. *Collaboration* refers to two or more people working together to achieve some common purpose or shared goal. The end result of collaborative learning is a product of the group, to which each individual has contributed his or her own special skills or talents. In fieldwork, collaborative learning may involve two or more students working with one clinical supervisor or several fieldwork educators working with one or more students. Collaboration in fieldwork education also can refer to the multiple stakeholders involved in the process—faculty, academic fieldwork coordinators, fieldwork educators, practitioners, and students. Peters and Armstrong (1998) defined *collaborative learning* as "a special type of teaching and learning in which participants engage in co-construction of new knowledge. . . . Collaboration means that people labor together in order to construct something that did not exist before the collaboration" (p. 1). At least one study reported in the occupational therapy literature examined collaborative learning involving occupational therapists and occupational therapy assistants (Jung, Sainsbury, Grum, Wilkins, & Tryssenaar, 2002). A study in the physical therapy literature demonstrated that clinical competence was enhanced following use of the collaborative learning model (DeClute & Ladyshewsky, 1993).

Some educators use the terms *cooperative learning* and *collaborative learning* interchangeably; however, the two terms imply different concepts. Cooperative learning "involves learners working together at the level of giving advice and help, sharing resources, swapping ideas or techniques. It does not involve exploring problems at a deeper level" (Cross et al., 2006, p. 78). Students or practitioners work together on a common task or tasks, providing mutual support and sharing resources. But the teacher or supervisor retains control; he or she assigns the tasks to be learned, starts and stops the group learning activity, and monitors how students are doing. Collaborative learning, on the other hand,

> involves a genuine desire and active interest in identifying and solving problems jointly. Inherent in this approach is commitment to assisting fellow learners, as far as possible, to achieve their own learning goals as well as the goals of the group. (Cross et al., 2006, p. 78)

Collaborative learning is based on a different epistemology from cooperative learning, that of Vgotsky and social constructivism. Vygotsky's theories emphasize social relationships and suggest that learning occurs through group interaction when the group participants exchange ideas and are exposed to the different perspectives of the other participants. Motivation to learn is increased when group members work toward a commonly held goal. Success comes to the entire group, not just the individual learner.

When people work together in a collaborative manner, they have to negotiate certain issues if they are to accomplish their tasks. These issues include authority, group membership roles, control of tasks and progress, values, and norms. Through resolving these issues, the group members arrive at a body of socially constructed knowledge. Teachers and students work together to create new knowledge and/or new meaning. The teacher is a co-learner in the process rather than the "expert"; he or she is as much an active participant as the students, but the teacher's role is to facilitate the learning process. Learners are held accountable not only for their own learning but also for the learning of their peers. In the process, they learn important teamwork skills that will be valued when they enter the workforce.

Education psychologist David W. Johnson and research Robert T. Johnson (quoted in Cohn, Dooley, & Simmons, 2001) articulated the following principles of collaborative learning:

> Knowledge is constructed, discovered, transformed, and extended by students. The educator creates a setting where students, when given a subject, can explore, question, research, interpret, and solidify the knowledge they feel is important.
>
> Students actively construct their own knowledge. Students guided by the educator actively seek out new knowledge.
>
> Education is a personal transformation among students and between educators and students as they work together.
>
> All of the above can only take place within a cooperative context. There is no competition among students to strive to be better than the other. Students take responsibility for each other's learning. (p. 71)

Occupational therapists Ellen S. Cohn, Nancy Robert Dooley, and Lynn A. Simmons (2001), in an outstanding article on collaborative fieldwork, described the five conditions that Johnson and colleagues (1991) identified as basic to collaborative learning:

> *Positive interdependence:* A recognition by group members that they are linked together in a way that none of them can be successful unless they all are. Students must believe they sink or swim together. Within every cooperative task, students develop mutual learning goals.
>
> *Face-to-face interaction*: Group members have access to each other's talents and resources and promote each other's success. Students interact to help each other accomplish a task.
>
> *Individual accountability*: Requires each group member to be active, learn, and be able to do things that they learned in the group. Students team together so they can subsequently perform at a higher level as individuals. Students are held accountable for their share of the work.
>
> *Cooperative skills*: Need to be encouraged and taught as carefully as the subject matter.
>
> *Group processing*: Students in cooperative relationships need to process their experiences on an ongoing basis to become more skillful in working as a group. Fieldwork educators need to ensure

that members of the group discuss how well they are achieving goals and maintaining effective working relationships. Group members need to identify what is helpful or non-helpful. (p. 72)

To implement a collaborative fieldwork model with a group of students, the fieldwork educator and the students must understand the nature of collaborative learning. I usually assign students articles to read, such as Cohn et al. (2001), so that they understand that cooperation, rather than competition, is the goal. The fieldwork educator must take care not to single out students for individual achievements or accomplishments. Rather, the group as a whole must get regular feedback on how well they are working together as group.

The collaborative model works very well when the fieldwork educator cannot be with the students all the time, although this is not its primary purpose. Students need to be directed to provide each other feedback after observing each other perform interventions. The fieldwork educator needs to give up some of the control he or she may have had in more traditional fieldwork situations. In accordance with collaborative learning principles, the educator is not the expert and takes on more of a facilitative role than a teacher role. The pay-off is students who develop strong team values, can function more autonomously, and become more self-directed.

 Learning Activities

1. Think back to the first time you used reflection as a learning activity. Describe what the learning context was and how reflection enhanced your learning. What kind of reflective activities did you use (Brown & Ryan, 2000, p. 122)?

2. What does *reflective practice* mean to you? Write down your definition (Brown & Ryan, 2000, p. 122).

3. Think about a professional experience you would like to explore to further your learning. Use the following questions to guide the process (Brown & Ryan, 2000, p. 124):

   • Go back to the experience you had. What happened? Describe it.
   • Pay attention to the feelings you are having now as you reflect on the experience. How did you feel at the time?

- Now re-evaluate the experience. How did the experience happen? What does it make you think about? What conclusions does this reflection lead you to? How do you make sense of what happened as you now reflect on the experience?

4. Think of a time when you were a supervisor. Did you actively engage supervisees in reflective thinking? How did you encourage that? What worked well? What didn't work so well? What can you do next time or try differently so that you are better able to elicit reflective thinking in your supervisees?

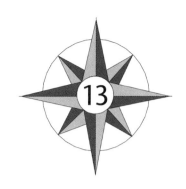

Training Issues in Clinical Supervision

In any educational program the most important single factor of success is the instructor. The satisfaction and effectiveness of the students in their clinical practice experience, as well as many of their future attitudes toward their work, will depend almost entirely upon the quality of supervision. In addition to a broad knowledge of the subject, and certain personal traits, it is essential that the teaching supervisor have a liking for and a degree of skills in teaching.

(Whitcomb, 1951, p. 129)

The issue of training for supervisors has appeared in the literature for decades not only in occupational therapy but also in psychology, nursing, social work, counseling, physical therapy, audiology, and other fields. Recommendations related to training, credentialing, and/or certification for occupational therapy fieldwork educators date back to at least 1931. That year saw the development of the "Minimum Standards for Courses of Training in Occupational Therapy" by the newly formed American Occupational Therapy Association (AOTA). According to these standards, "the hospital-practice training of students must be supervised by a properly qualified, registered occupational therapist, who is not only competent in her department, but has shown ability to handle students-in-training" (quoted in Quiroga, 1995, p. 230).

The first mention of the need for formalized training for fieldwork educators was in a paper presented by E. Mary MacDonald, the principal of Dorset House School of Occupational Therapy in Oxford, England, at the Fifth International Congress of the World Federation of Occupational Therapy in Zurich in 1970. At that meeting, MacDonald (1971) stated,

> Courses for clinical supervisors should be developed on formal lines. They should ultimately lead to a certificate for an adequate 3-month course or, perhaps, by an aggregation of certificates of attendance at 2 or 3 courses over a period of several years, ultimately leading to incremental recognition. They could be organized by the Professional Training Board and the schools, in collaboration.

In 1987, the Representative Assembly of AOTA charged the Commission on Education to explore alternative Level II fieldwork models, and in 1989 the

Final Report of the Fieldwork Study Committee was issued. Appendix A formally addressed the need for fieldwork supervision:

> Qualification and preparation of fieldwork supervisors have repeatedly been expressed as concerns of both clinical settings and academic programs. Certification of sites and/or supervisors has been proposed in the past but not implemented. Nevertheless, the need for more formalized preparation of fieldwork supervisors persists. The fact remains that fieldwork supervisors are clinical educators who must be apprised of educational content and technology to function competently. Clinical educators are indispensable in acculturating occupational therapy students and shaping clinical reasoning. Responsibility for preparing clinical educators for the role of fieldwork supervisor must be shared by academic programs, clinical settings, and the national association. . . . *If we value competent fieldwork supervision, we must invest resources and recognize the accomplishment.* (Opacich, quoted in Privott, 1998, p. 419; italics added for emphasis).

A special issue of the *American Journal of Occupational Therapy* published in February 1995 was devoted to fieldwork issues, and occupational therapist Karin Opacich (1995) succinctly framed the issues:

> Having the opportunity to sift through the AOTA archives reminds one that unless the full scope and impact of a problem is perceived and addressed, it tends to re-emerge until it commands the attention it deserves. Adequacy of fieldwork sites (number and quality) is such an issue; another is the preparation of fieldwork supervisors. . . . Some occupational therapists have questioned the fairness and the wisdom of expecting clinical programs and practitioners to design and provide education in clinical settings for which they are usually not formally prepared. . . . Supervising students necessitates a commitment to acquiring some additional competencies to most positively affect students' career paths and choices. (p. 161)

Need for Clinical Supervisor Training

Learning to become a clinical supervisor is both an art and a science. The learner can read many books and articles, but reading will be insufficient for learning; an experiential component needs to be built into the training process. Hawkins and Shohet (2000) suggested a process that is illustrated in Figure 13.1. What is particularly interesting about this suggested process is that it makes use of multiple methods: "It is grossly inadequate just to send them on a short

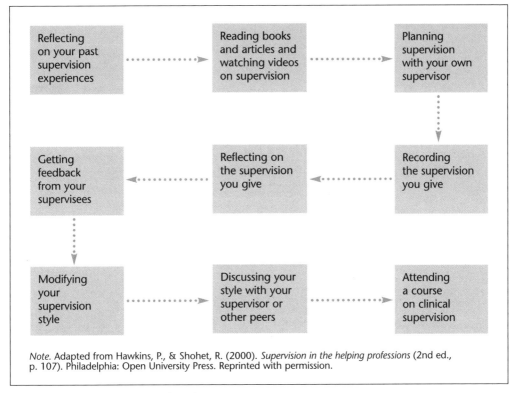

Note. Adapted from Hawkins, P., & Shohet, R. (2000). *Supervision in the helping professions* (2nd ed., p. 107). Philadelphia: Open University Press. Reprinted with permission.

FIGURE 13.1. The supervision learning process.

supervisor training course and then expect them to function well as a supervisor" (p. 79).

When I give supervision workshops, I often start with a case example. Gandy (2002), a physical therapist, described a situation that is all too common: A practitioner with one year of experience is told that she will be getting her first student shortly. The center coordinator of clinical education provided minimal if any guidance, which resulted in Gandy reaching a state of near panic and reflection on her inadequacies to begin providing clinical supervision:

The center coordinator asked me if I had any questions. After a brief pause, I quietly replied, "No." Not only did I not know where to begin to ask the first question, but also I was absolutely overwhelmed by the responsibility. I assumed that everyone who was assigned a student after 1 year of practice must be capable of serving as a clinical instructor, and I did not want to respond any differently than my peers.

Afterwards, I realized that in 1 week I would be responsible for the student's clinical learning experience and had not a clue as to how to structure a planned experience. At least I was familiar with the student evaluation instrument because I had used the same instrument when I was a student. I had no experience providing a student orientation before and had only completed a new employee orientation. In reality, I knew very little about teaching students in the clinic other than my recollections of being a student in the clinic and some classroom lectures I vaguely remembered on patient education and clinical education. I also tried to reflect on what my [supervisor] did during my clinical experiences. For the next week I tried to informally question more experienced . . . therapists about how they taught their students. I did not want them to know that I felt incompetent. . . . What did I remember most about my clinical educators that were positive or negative? Based on my limited discussions with professional peers and my personal reflections, I developed a better, albeit limited, understanding of my perceived roles and responsibilities. All too soon it was time for me to teach my first student. (pp. 211–212)

Sound familiar? Although this narrative was written by a physical therapist, it could just as easily have been written by an occupational therapy practitioner. In the early days of occupational therapy, clinical education was based on the apprenticeship model, in which the supervisor took a student under his or her wing and showed the student everything he or she knew. But the apprenticeship model has limited utility in the current health care climate, where entry-level practitioners have to demonstrate independent clinical reasoning skills and problem-solving skills. Christie (1999) articulated her belief that occupational therapy practitioners need to learn more about the conceptual base of supervision to both provide and receive effective supervision, but as Sweeney, Webley, and Treacher (2001a, 2001b) wrote, supervision has received minimal attention in the occupational therapy literature:

This paucity of exploration stems from an assumption (which permeates the literature on supervision) that expertise as a clinician implies expertise as a supervisor. However, there is no empirical evidence to support this implication and, indeed, there is evidence to support the opposite claim: that supervisors are advised not to respond to their supervisees as they would to a patient, that the skills inherent in being a supervisor partially overlap with the skills necessary to be a clinician but are somewhat different, and that the senior clinician may not be able to remember what it is like to be a novice. (Sweeney et al., 2001a, pp. 337–338)

Higgs and McAllister (2005) noted the consequences of lack of training for clinical educators in the health professions:

> Clinical educators lack an explicit theoretical and philosophical framework for their educational activities, myths about clinical education are pervasive, integration of academic and clinical curricula suffers, and there is a mismatch between the theory and the practice of clinical education. (p. 156)

In the same vein, Strohschein, Hagler, and May (2002) articulated the pressing need for changes in the way clinical education is provided:

> Contributing to what we believe is an inconsistency of approach is inadequate preparation of clinicians for the important and complex role of clinical educator. Expertise in clinical practice does not imply expertise in clinical education. . . . Because those clinical educators lacked formal education in this area, they often learned the role primarily by trial and error. . . . We argue that there are many excellent clinical educators and positive clinical education experiences, but at the present this may be due more to clinicians' intuition and natural abilities as educators than to their effective, consistent approach to the clinical education process. (pp. 162, 171)

Suggested Structure of Training in Clinical Supervision

The structure of a course or training program for fieldwork educators can take many forms depending on the learning needs and time frames available. The following list outlines the topical areas that need to be addressed in a training curriculum:

- *Overview of supervision:* definitions of supervision, qualities of effective supervision, history of supervision in fieldwork education, purpose of supervision, and the expectations and skills of clinical educators
- *Learning about learning:* definition of androgogy, importance of learning in fieldwork education as an extension of the curriculum, adult learning theories, learning styles, use of Bloom's taxonomy in formulating behavioral objectives, and experiential learning cycles
- *Process of supervision:* functions of supervision, models of supervision, formats for supervision (individual, group, peer, team, collaborative,

remote, audiotaped or videotaped, and virtual), reflective practice, and supervision styles.

- *Skills of clinical supervisors:* communication, feedback, listening, development and maintenance of relationships, openness to learning, ethical conduct, multicultural competence, legal issues, confidentiality, and flexibility.
- *Supervisor's toolbox:* learning contracts, supervision contracts, supervisory session notes, self-assessment of supervisory skills and competencies, professional development plan, evaluation of supervisee competencies, supervisees' evaluations of supervisor, self-care skills, and supervision for the supervisor.
- *Typical problems in supervision:* discussion of problems supervisors encounter with supervisees, ways to apply theories and concepts to practice, and discussion or role-playing of sample situations (proposed by either the instructor or the supervisors). Typical problems include the following:
  - Personality conflicts or disagreements in the supervisory relationship
  - Supervisees' overdependence on the supervisor
  - Supervisees' fear of calculated risks in the learning process
  - Supervisees' anxiety
  - Supervisees' lack of preparation for supervisory sessions
  - Supervisees' invitation to "grab a cup of coffee"
  - Supervisees' failure to follow established policies or to modify behavior based on the supervisor's recommendations
  - Supervisees' difficult questions—which to respond to directly, which to avoid, and which require further probing by the supervisor to facilitate reflective practice
  - Supervisees' need for constant praise and positive reinforcement
  - Supervisors' feelings of insecurity
  - Supervisees' blaming themselves for failures in clients' treatment
  - Supervisees' or supervisors' feelings of romantic attraction to the other
  - Supervisees' lack of progress toward achieving learning objectives
  - Differences between supervisors and supervisees in age, gender, academic degree, culture, religion, values, and so forth
  - Supervisees' crying when given negative feedback
  - Supervisees' failing fieldwork at the midterm evaluation.

Each topical area should include a balance of didactic and experiential learning activities and group and individual activities. Multiple media may include video clips on supervision sessions, electronic slide presentations, presentations of didactic materials, lecture, and interactive learning activities. Training workshops should be broken up into shorter sessions; in the interim between sessions, participants can go back to their work sites to use the material learned and then return to training with examples. In addition, supervisors should produce a videotape of a supervisory session for review by their own supervisor or trainer or someone who can objectively assess the quality of their supervision.

In addition to offering this training course to occupational therapy practitioners, some of the proposed content should be provided to students before they graduate from their educational programs. In this way, students will be better prepared to use supervision effectively. In addition, because practitioners with one year of experience can begin supervising students, it makes sense to introduce students to the concepts underlying the theory and practice of clinical supervision.

Role Development of Clinical Supervisors

Completing a course on clinical supervision is not the end of the learning process for supervisors, just as graduation from an educational program is not the end of learning process for occupational therapy practitioners. There is a definite progression in the role development of clinical supervisors, and several theories of role development have been proposed.

Psychiatrist Paul Rodenhauser (1994), for example, conceptualized four separate stages of supervisor development:

1. In the *emulation stage,* new supervisors tend initially to emulate their previous role models, providing a foundation for helping them gain confidence.
2. In the *conceptualization stage,* supervisors engage in dialogue with peers to discover new methods and ways of doing things.
3. The *incorporation stage* occurs when supervisors begin to recognize how important the supervisory relationship is and become more sensitive to the impact they have on their supervisees.
4. In the *consolidation stage,* supervisors begin to integrate their knowledge and experience.

The integrated development model (IDM; Stoltenberg, McNeill, & Delworth, 1998) outlined three stages of supervisory development:

- *Level 1* supervisors want to provide supervision correctly and may experience anxiety.
- *Level 2* supervisors experience confusion and conflict, and most of their focus is on the supervisee; they now understand that

supervision is more complex and difficult than they thought it would be.

- *Level 3* supervisors function with autonomy and use their own supervision to advance their supervisory skills. Level 3 supervisors often become master supervisors, able to supervise any student or supervisee with ease.

In describing the supervisor complexity model, psychologist C. Edward Watkins (1990) theorized that several development issues are central to a supervisor's development—competency versus incompetence, autonomy versus dependency, identity versus identity diffusion, and self-awareness versus unawareness. The Watkins model includes four stages:

- *Stage 1* is role shock. New supervisors feel that they are "playing" the role of a supervisor and may feel like an imposter. They cope by imposing rules and a somewhat rigid structure and maintaining distance from their supervisees.
- *Stage 2* is role recovery and transition. Supervisors at this stage begin to develop their own supervisory identity as their confidence increases. They can assess their own strengths and weaknesses more accurately, but they still experience fluctuations in their self-assessment of their abilities, sometimes feeling good about how they supervise others and sometimes feeling inadequate.
- *Stage 3* is role consolidation. In this stage, supervisors have become more consistent in their reflections about their ability to supervise. They exert less control when supervising and are able to express more support and encouragement to their supervisees.
- *Stage 4* is role mastery. Supervisors at this stage are consistent in their approach toward supervisees, even when the abilities of those supervisees vary widely. Their sense of a supervisory self is integrated with a balance between theoretical knowledge and their own style of supervision.

The Hess (1986) model conceptualizes three stages in the supervisor development process:

1. The beginning stage, in which the new supervisor makes the transition from novice to supervisor, experiences role ambiguity, and is unsure of his or her teaching abilities;
2. The exploration stage, characterized by alternation between the extremes of being too restrictive and too intrusive with supervisees; and
3. Confirmation of the supervisor identity, the stage at which supervisors begin to feel a sense of gratification and pride when their super-

visees succeed; at this stage, supervisors are less dependent on others for praise and validation and are able to be fully present in the supervisory relationship.

Psychologist Anne Alonso (1983) outlined a model influenced by both the psychodynamic and life span development perspectives. She described the developmental stages as having three themes: (1) self and identity, (2) relationship between the supervisor and the therapist, and (3) relationship between the supervisor and the administrative structure of supervisor's workplace. Alonso identified three stages in a supervisor's development:

1. In the *novice stage,* supervisors are

   nurturing a dream about what they might become, but also are confronted with developing a sense of self-as-supervisor. They must also cope with the anxiety that comes from needing to deal with narcissistic developmental needs (i.e., for validation, for approval, and for role models) that emerge in response to the need to defend themselves as novices once again after already having achieved some sense of mastery as therapists. (Bernard & Goodyear, 2004, p. 280).

2. In the *midcareer stage,* supervisors become mentors to others as they shift the focus away from themselves and toward others.

3. In the *late career stage,* supervisors struggle to maintain their sense of professional self-esteem as younger colleagues begin to advance in their careers and ageism results in devaluation of older professionals in the workplace.

The Dreyfus model of skill acquisition was originally developed by Hubert Dreyfus, a mathematician, who studied the process of skill acquisition in chess players, Air Force pilots, and Army tank drivers and commanders (cited in Benner, 2004, p. 188). Patricia Benner, a nurse, adapted the model to study the professional development of nurses, and the application can serve occupational therapists and occupational therapy assistants as well. The five levels or stages of skill in the Dreyfus model as follows:

- *Level 1, novice:* In the first level, the individual is still in school, learning the knowledge and skills for professional practice. The focus is on the immediate skills at hand and on getting them right.

- *Level 2, advanced beginner:* New graduates in entry-level practice are advanced beginners; they rely heavily on feedback from others and may be quite anxious in new situations. Such practitioners

  have a level of trust in the environment and in the legitimacy of co-workers' knowledge, which allows them to absorb information as fact. This trust sets up qualities of freedom and exhilaration in learning that are probably only available to those who do not yet comprehend the contingent nature of both the situation and what is known about it. The freedom in learning is furthered because advanced beginners do not yet feel responsible for managing clinical situations with which they are unfamiliar. (p. 192)

- *Level 3, competent:* Practitioners with 1 to 2 years of practice are at this stage. Their clinical competence with patients is uneven, dependent on their experience with that population. They do more planning and seek to apply their knowledge to new situations, which minimizes their anxiety.
- *Level 4, proficient:* This stage is characterized by growing proficiency in clinical situations, and practitioners are able to synthesize the meaning of a patient's responses. They are accountable and intuitive and highly skilled. When in unfamiliar situations, they still refer to guidelines.
- *Level 5, expert:* Benner labeled this stage "practical wisdom" (p. 196). Expert practitioners are able to rapidly assess new situations and can move into action quickly:

> Based on enriched experiential learning spawned by increasing ability to read the current situation in terms of their deep familiarity with similar and dissimilar situations, nurses develop a sense of whether they have a good (better or poorer) grasp of the situation. Skilled know-how now allows for more fluid and rapid performance of procedures. (p. 197)

Research on Outcomes of Training for Supervisory Competence

It is not surprising that there has been little research on the outcomes of training for supervisory competence, although such research is beginning to emerge. Some studies have described the impact of gaining supervisory skills and knowledge. For example, Vendrely and Carter (2004) focused on the impact of formal training on evaluations of students' performance, demonstrating an improvement in the ability to assess skills. Another study by Hook and Lawson-Porter (2003) examined the outcomes of interdisciplinary training and showed that there are core skills in supervision that can be effectively taught across disciplines. MacKenzie, Zakrzewski, Walter, and McCluskey (2001) described a collaborative workshop taught by four educational programs in Australia that included discussion of the foci and philosophy of their curricula in addition to teaching of supervisory skills. The authors assessed the reasons why fieldwork educators attended this workshop, and the most frequently cited were "I want to do a better job than my supervisor did when I was a student" and "I need help making the placement worthwhile for me as a supervisor" (MacKenzie et al., 2001, p. 6). Other reasons cited were the need to upgrade supervisory skills, to gain an understanding of educational programs, and to develop a professional support network.

One of the most significant studies was reported by Milne and James (2002) in the psychology field. Following extensive interviews and observations, they identified several supervisory behaviors and measured them before and after a formalized training program. The supervisory behaviors they identified included managing; listening; supporting; summarizing; providing feedback; gathering information; checking supervisees' theoretical knowledge base; challenging; informing and educating; guiding experiential learning, modeling, and role-play; self-disclosing; disagreeing; doing video observation; and engaging in other behaviors such as documentation, social conversation, and setting up equipment. Supervisee behaviors were identified as reflecting, experimenting, conceptualizing, experiencing emotion, planning, and engaging in other behaviors, including paperwork and other assignments and social conversation. The authors organized the supervisory and supervisee behaviors into an experiential learning model based on Kolb's (1984) experiential learning cycle. They measured the number of identified behaviors in supervisors who participated in formal training and those who had had no training and demonstrated that training increased both the number of supervisory behaviors and the ability to facilitate an increased number of supervisee behaviors. Readers are encouraged to obtain this article and to use its findings in their practice.

That training increases competence in clinical supervisors has been repeatedly demonstrated in the fields of social work, nursing, psychology, mental health counseling, and physical therapy. Each of these professions is in varying stages of development in creating formal training programs. As Fidler (1966) observed four decades ago,

> In order for a profession to fulfill its obligations to the society it serves, learning must be a continuing, ongoing process. Education for the profession must not stop at the time of graduation. We must teach in such a way that learning will result in a research attitude; a way of thinking so that questioning, investigation and constructively critical evaluation becomes a way of life and thus learning and growth a continuing process. (p. 8)

Learning Activities

1. Even if you have already supervised others, imagine for a moment that supervision is very new to you and that you have just agreed to begin providing clinical supervision to someone. Reflect on the question, What do I want to get out of being a supervisor (van Ooijen, 2000, p. 80)?

2. Imagine that you have just agreed to begin supervising a group of four Level II fieldwork students starting next week. How do you feel about this? How do you feel about your skills, abilities, preparation, and so forth? Portray how you feel on a large sheet of blank paper, in whatever way you wish, using markers, colored pencils, or crayons (van Ooijen, 2000, p. 105).

3. Design a fieldwork educator course that would meet your learning needs at this time. What would you change in designing a course to train students in supervision? What would you change in providing advanced workshops for experienced supervisors?

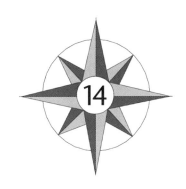

Clinical Supervision in Role-Emerging Practice Settings

If occupational therapists are to take leadership roles in community programs, training must begin at the student level. Curricula should include courses in description and assessment of community needs and resources, systems theory, and program development.

(Grossman, 1974, p. 591)

Occupational therapy fieldwork education has been expanding into different practice settings for decades as practitioners have explored different venues for providing both occupational therapy services and unique learning opportunities for students. The occupational therapy literature has given these settings different names, including *nontraditional, role-emerging, alternative,* and *independent* community settings. The term *nontraditional* seems to have fallen out of favor; what is nontraditional may become traditional or mainstream within a few years. *Role-emerging* appears to be the most frequently used term currently, but Mulholland and Derdall (2005) suggested that it implies the development of a paid position for an occupational therapist, which may or may not happen; these Canadian fieldwork educators preferred the term *independent community placement. Role-emerging,* however, is the way fieldwork in these settings is referred to in the Accreditation Council for Occupational Therapy Education (ACOTE) standards, and I use it in this chapter, which presents some of the common threads of these type of opportunities, focusing on the skills fieldwork educators need to maximize student learning outcomes.

History of Role-Emerging Fieldwork

The occupational therapy literature is full of descriptions of innovative programs that were designed with the dual purposes of expanding occupational therapy services to a previously unserved population and meeting the ever-increasing demand for fieldwork sites. Some of these programs were developed primarily in response to a community need, whereas others were developed primarily out of a need for fieldwork sites. Occupational therapy researcher and professor Sharon A. Cermak (1976) developed a service–learning program to provide early intervention services to children and their families in a local day care center. The students, from Boston University, provided perceptual–motor activities to the children, screened the children for developmental delays, and provided educational workshops for their parents. In that same year, Cromwell and Kielhofner (1976) reported on a program developed out of the University of Southern California in which students learned program development skills in designing and implementing several community-based programs.

Menks, Sittler, Weaver, and Yannow (1977) from the University of Florida developed a program for elderly individuals with mental illness consisting of outreach services and activity groups. Platt, Martell, and Clements (1977) from Eastern Michigan University reported on a Level I mental health fieldwork placement at a federal correctional institution. Drake (1995) reported on a day care program for homeless children that served as a Level I fieldwork placement for students at the University of Alabama at Birmingham. Faculty from the University of Kentucky (Rydeen, Kautzmann, Cowan, & Benzing, 1995) developed community-based programs in response to a shortage of Level I fieldwork placements in rural areas in the areas of pediatrics, mental health, homelessness, and adult day care for people with Alzheimer's disease. One of these projects—a homeless shelter—evolved into a Level II fieldwork placement (Shorndike & Howell, 2001). Faculty from Washington University developed a community practice division in 1995 that addressed service, education, and research. Students worked alongside faculty in a variety of community projects, including homeless shelters, residential centers for children, early childhood or day care centers, community mental health programs, meal programs for senior citizens, community work settings, and many more. Students had the opportunity to do their Level I fieldwork at these program sites, and some returned to complete their master's-degree research projects. Gabarini and Pearlman (1998) described the use of home health care as an innovative fieldwork alternative.

Recently, four articles in the occupational therapy literature described the development of community-based programs uniting academic faculty, occupational therapy practitioners, and students in a model known as a practice–scholar program. Suarez-Balcazar and colleagues (2005) from the University of Illinois at Chicago described their university–community partnership in two unique programs, one a domestic violence shelter and the other an independent living center. Although students participated in these programs, the primary objective was to engage in a university–community partnership for participatory action research. Faculty from Duquesne University described a collaboration with a county jail in a community reintegration project (Crist, Fairman, et al., 2005) and an academic–practice partnership with several other community sites, including day care centers and homeless shelters (Crist, Munoz, Hansen, Benson, & Provident, 2005). Miller and Johnson (2005) reported on a partnership program between faculty members from Thomas Jefferson University, master clinicians, and students in providing services at a number of community sites, including homeless shelters, senior centers, assisted-living facilities, community mental health programs, and sheltered workshops.

Fieldwork in Role-Emerging Settings

There is a common element in most of the articles cited in the preceding section—that of providing high-quality, challenging fieldwork placements to students where they will be able to apply what they have learned in the classroom to real-life practice. The purpose of fieldwork is to prepare entry-level practitioners for the workforce. But occupational therapy practitioners of today are different from those who were trained in the first 50 to 60 years of the profession. Gone are the large numbers of jobs in state psychiatric hospitals and the large occupational therapy departments in hospitals and rehabilitation centers as the shift in health care has moved occupational therapy services to community-based and home-based settings. Today's occupational therapy practitioner must know not only how to work with people suffering from diseases, illnesses, and injuries but also how to design and develop programs, manage resources, provide educational services, research treatment outcomes, obtain funding for services, and advocate for clients as well as professional issues. As Baptiste (2005) observed, "Without question the environment around us has broader and grander expectations of us as practitioners than in the past" (p. 179).

In many instances, educational programs developed role-emerging sites when enrollment in their programs increased and existing fieldwork placements were too few. When placements have worked to the mutual advantage of the community-based agency and the student, some agencies have created a full- or part-time occupational therapy position. What educational programs have discovered in the process is the benefit to students in terms of improved learning outcomes, increased clinical reasoning skills, and increased ability to problem solve. Thus, role-emerging practice placements have provided opportunities to students that more traditional placements have not been able to provide. Sullivan and Finlayson (2000) observed,

> For many of these students, the current "apprentice" model of fieldwork supervision does not allow them to really "stretch their wings" and to assume almost full responsibility for their learning experiences. Role-emerging fieldwork can offer these students the "just-right" challenge, and help them to gain confidence and competence to practice in new and innovative settings. (p. 13)

Some role-emerging practice is associated with the development of practice–scholar programs involving partnerships between academic faculty and community-based practitioners. Both parties work together in a collaborative manner, and fieldwork students greatly benefit from the unique mentoring opportunities. Learning about role-emerging practice in a classroom and reading articles about it is a vastly different educational experience from learning about role-emerging practice through active participation in this model. These collaborative programs usually start with Level I fieldwork students and then gradually add Level II fieldwork students. But role-emerging practice accomplishes another goal—that of bringing the occupational therapy profession closer to the *Centennial Vision* outlined by the American Occupational Therapy Association (AOTA) (2006): "We envision that occupational therapy is a powerful, widely recognized, science-driven, and globally connected and diverse workforce meeting society's occupational needs."

Role-Emerging Areas of Occupational Therapy Practice

AOTA former Vice President and occupational scientist Charles Christiansen identified 10 areas of role-emerging practice:

1. Ergonomics consulting
2. Design and accessibility consulting and home modifications
3. Older driver assessment and training
4. Consulting to assisted-living facilities
5. Technology and assistive-device development and consulting
6. Health and wellness consulting
7. Low-vision rehabilitation
8. Alzheimer's disease care and caregiver training
9. Needs of children and youths
10. Community services.

Required Knowledge and Skills for Practicing in the Community

Occupational therapist Mary Ann McColl (1998) wrote about the knowledge and skills that students and practitioners need to provide services in the community. In terms of knowledge, she suggested that occupational therapy practitioners need coursework in cultural anthropology, sociology, organizational psychology, economics, business management, epidemiology, public health, politics, policy, systems theory, and history. In addition, McColl wrote that practitioners and students need to be able to respond to the following questions:

- What is a community?
- How do organizations and communities develop?
- Who governs organizations and communities, and how?
- What are the community's resources, where are they, and how do their members gain access to them?
- How does one assess the needs of the community?
- How can one be a catalyst or agent of change?
- How do people with disabilities live in the community?
- What barriers and obstacles exist in the community that prevent people with disabilities from full inclusion and participation?

- How do people in the community develop and pursue their chosen occupations? What occupations are popular in this community?

Scott (2000) suggested that students assigned to role-emerging fieldwork settings need to be able to work both collaboratively with others and independently, to come up with creative solutions to problems, to understand what is meant by *consultation* and be able to use a consultative approach, and to work cooperatively with peers who are also assigned to the fieldwork site. Sullivan and Finlayson (2000) suggested that faculty should select students on the basis of a very careful assessment of whether they can meet the demands of the setting. Students must demonstrate a self-directed approach to learning, and those who have had difficulties in their previous fieldwork placements should not be selected for fieldwork in role-emerging settings. The authors further stated that students selected must demonstrate their ability to take responsibility for their own learning:

> A role-emerging fieldwork placement requires a great deal of work, and a strong commitment is required on the part of the student. Therefore this step of the selection process involves assessing the student's comprehension of the learning opportunities, risks and benefits, and ability to articulate potential linkages between OT philosophy, core concepts, and practice opportunities at his/her setting of choice. (p. 14)

Supervisory Skills Needed in Role-Emerging Practice Areas

ACOTE (2007) has written standards for educational programs to follow regarding the supervision of fieldwork students. The current standards were adopted in 1998, and a new set of standards were recently adopted that go into effect January 1, 2008. These standards define role-emerging fieldwork settings as those that do not employ occupational therapy practitioners and specify that fieldwork educators must have at least 3 years of professional work experience as an occupational therapist or occupational therapy assistant and 6 hours of supervision per week before beginning to supervise fieldwork students in such settings. This standard goes into effect in 2008 and includes a 2-hour increase over the previous requirement of supervision per week. This more rigorous standard is essential, because supervision in role-emerging practice settings is an advanced practice skill requiring additional competencies in population-based assessment and treatment, consultation, distance supervision, collaboration with professionals from other disciplines, and student evaluation skills.

The standards also specify that there be a documented plan for supervision; supervision must initially be direct but then may decrease over time as the students' skills increase. What is essential is that students have adequate opportunities for role modeling: Students should have opportunities to observe their occupational therapy supervisor work with clients, and supervisors must observe students working with clients. The standards specify that supervisors be available at all times to students during working hours, but this requirement can be met through a variety of modalities—phone, e-mail, pager, fax, and so forth. In addition, someone from another profession must be available onsite to the student during working hours. Ideally, this person should be familiar with the scope of occupational therapy practice and the kinds of services students can and cannot provide.

What kinds of supervisory practices have been demonstrated to work in role-emerging practice settings? In my two decades of providing supervision to students in such settings, I have learned much about what works and what does not. Students must understand the structure of the fieldwork placement. They need to know when they will see the supervisor and how often and to have all of the supervisor's emergency contact numbers. Students need to know that they can call the supervisor whenever, for whatever reason. I state this very clearly up front to reassure students that I am always available to them and that contacting me is not a sign of failure—that's what I'm there for. I give students my office phone number, my cell phone number, my home telephone number, and both of my e-mail addresses. There also needs to be a backup plan, so another professional is assigned to be available to students when I am not onsite.

In my experience, it is essential to articulate my supervision model to students and to give them reading assignments to help them understand it better. I currently use a collaborative learning model in my part-time position as an occupational therapy consultant in an acute psychiatric inpatient unit in a general hospital. My site accepts students from multiple schools, and I supervise between 2 and 4 students at any given time. In the past I have successfully used the collaborative learning model in other community-based mental health settings, such as clubhouse programs, psychiatric rehabilitation programs, day treatment programs, residential programs, and prevocational programs.

On the first day of their fieldwork assignment, I explain to students what I mean by a *collaborative learning model* and assign them an article (Cohn, 2001) as their first reading. I make sure they understand that collaborative learning is more than just group supervision, that it involves the co-construction of new knowledge and the investment of all students in each other's learning, and that the success of one becomes the success of all. I set up a structure for the students to sit down together after each group intervention to discuss how the intervention went and provide each other with feedback on their group facilitation skills. I assign group projects to further advance the idea of their working together toward a common goal.

After I have explained my approach to collaborative learning, I provide a structure for students' learning in the form of a 12-week outline of assignments. Students are relieved greatly by having a written structure; it allays their anxiety over what they will do during the Level II fieldwork. This list of assignments also reinforces that the placement is an occupational therapy learning experience; with role-emerging practice placements, students often are afraid that they will not get a "real" occupational therapy experience and that the experience will be more typical of the profession of their backup supervisor. This fear is more pronounced in community settings, where staff roles are typically somewhat blurred. The job of the occupational therapy fieldwork educator is to create mechanisms, assignments, and other learning activities that reinforce the role of occupational therapy in role-emerging practice. It also is essential that supervisors be onsite for sufficient time to provide students with opportunities to observe them working with clients and to directly observe students' therapeutic interventions with clients and give direct feedback. Students always value the occupational therapy supervisor's feedback more than that of their peers or an onsite supervisor from another profession.

Another factor in supervising students in role-emerging practice settings is the increased importance of students' active use of supervision. If the supervisor holds a weekly formal supervision session, students must come prepared to be active participants, bringing questions that arose during the week, cases to present and discuss, and written assignments to submit and review. If only group supervision is to be provided, the supervisor must make this clear to students and specify how they can obtain individual sessions. I provide opportunities for individual supervision via e-mail and require that students send me an e-mail at least once a week. To avoid the kinds of superficial messages that I have gotten in the past, I now require that students send me a "question of the week"; I often learn more about students' skills and abilities through the questions they ask than through their responses to my questions.

To elicit reflective thinking, I require students to keep a daily reflective journal in which they write about not what happened to them but how they felt about what happened and how they made sense of it. I assure students that they can write about anything, including any feelings (even negative ones) they have about me. I make it clear that I will read the journals and make comments on them but that no one else will see them. Whatever the ground rules are, the supervisor must state them up front. Previously, I allowed the onsite supervisor to also read students' journals, but there were several problems, so I discontinued the practice. The onsite supervisor may not understand the process and intent of reflective journaling, and he or she may have different expectations for the journal; any differences in approach are confusing to the student and ultimately counterproductive.

Supervisors must understand that no matter how much time they spend with students in role-emerging practice settings, the students probably will feel that it is not enough. Students assigned to role-emerging practice sites talk with their classmates in settings with a full-time occupational therapy supervisor, and they may perceive that site as the "better" placement. The supervisor should be prepared to articulate the advantages of role-emerging practice settings, including the opportunities they present to become more independent problem-solvers. I often assign other articles (e.g., Brown, 1998; Costa, 2007; Dour, Grey, & Michaelsen, 2007; Grimm & Massieon, 1998) to facilitate their understanding of the outcomes of their learning.

The payoff for supervisors is the immense pride they feel at what students accomplish over the 12 weeks and the opportunity to learn as much from students as the students learn from their supervisors. Supervision in role-emerging practice settings is a very student-centered experience, and the outcome is an occupational therapy practitioner with not only entry-level competencies in the specific practice area but also the ability to work independently, to critically self-evaluate their own work, to clearly articulate the role of occupational therapy, and to practice with increased clinical reasoning and problem-solving skills.

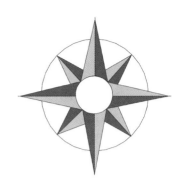

References and
Recommended Reading

Alonso, A. (1983). A developmental theory of psychodynamic supervision. *Clinical Supervisor, 1,* 23–26.

Accreditation Council for Occupational Therapy Education. (2007). *Accreditation standards for a master's-degree-level educational program for the occupational therapist.* Retrieved March 21, 2007, from www.aota.org/nu/docs/acotestandards 107.pdf.

American Medical Association. (1936). Essentials of an acceptable school of occupational therapy. Prepared by the Council of Medical Education and Hospitals of the American Medical Association. *Journal of the American Medical Association, 107,* 683–684.

American Medical Association. (1943). Essentials of an acceptable school of occupational therapy. Prepared by the Council of Medical Education and Hospitals of the American Medical Association. *Journal of the American Medical Association, 107,* 683–684.

American Occupational Therapy Association. (1924). *Archives of occupational therapy, 3.* Rockville, MD: Author.

American Occupational Therapy Association. (1948). *Manual for supervisors of student affiliations.* Rockville, MD: Author.

American Occupational Therapy Association. (1950). *A director's guide for a clinical training program for occupational therapy students.* Rockville, MD: Author.

American Occupational Therapy Association. (1965). *Guide book for an accredited curriculum in occupational therapy.* Rockville, MD: Author.

American Occupational Therapy Association. (1966a). *Manual for supervisors of student affiliations.* Rockville, MD: Author.

American Occupational Therapy Association. (1966b). *Student affiliations.* Dubuque, IA: William C. Brown.

American Occupational Therapy Association. (1971). Standards and guidelines of an occupational therapy affiliation program. *American Journal of Occupational Therapy, 25,* 314–316.

American Occupational Therapy Association. (1975). *Guidelines for developing a fieldwork experience program.* Rockville, MD: Author.

American Occupational Therapy Association. (1977). *Fieldwork experience manual for academic fieldwork coordinators, fieldwork supervisors, and students.* Rockville, MD: Author.

American Occupational Therapy Association. (1983a). Educational programs: Essentials of an accredited educational program for the occupational therapist. *American Journal of Occupational Therapy, 37,* 817–823.

American Occupational Therapy Association. (1983b). Educational programs: Essentials of an accredited educational program for the occupational therapy assistant. *American Journal of Occupational Therapy, 37,* 824–830.

American Occupational Therapy Association. (1984). *Fieldwork experience manual for academic fieldwork coordinators, fieldwork supervisors, and students.* Rockville, MD: Author.

American Occupational Therapy Association. (1991). *Self-paced instruction for clinical education and supervision.* Bethesda, MD: Author.

American Occupational Therapy Association. (1994). *Uniform terminology for occupational therapy* (3rd ed.). Bethesda, MD: Author.

American Occupational Therapy Association. (2000). *Meeting the fieldwork challenge.* Bethesda, MD: Author.

American Occupational Therapy Association. (2001). *Fieldwork experience assessment tool.* Retrieved March 23, 2007, from www.aota.org/nonmembers/area13/docs/feat.pdf.

American Occupational Therapy Association. (2002a). *Fieldwork performance evaluation forms—Occupational therapist.* Bethesda, MD: Author.

American Occupational Therapy Association. (2002b). *Fieldwork performance evaluation forms—Occupational therapy assistant.* Bethesda, MD: Author.

American Occupational Therapy Association. (2002c). *Occupational therapy practice framework: Domain and process.* Bethesda, MD: Author.

American Occupational Therapy Association. (2005a). Enforcement procedures for the *Occupational Therapy Code of Ethics. American Journal of Occupational Therapy, 59,* 643–652.

American Occupational Therapy Association. (2005b). Standards of practice for occupational therapists. *American Journal of Occupational Therapy, 59,* 663–665.

American Physical Therapy Association. (1997). *Physical therapy clinical instructor educator training manual.* Fairfax, VA: Author.

Ayers, W. (1986). About teaching and teachers. *Harvard Education Review, 56,* 49–51.

Bailey, D., & Schwartzberg, S. (2003). *Ethical and legal dilemmas in occupational therapy* (2nd ed.). Philadelphia: F. A. Davis.

Baltimore, M., & Crutchfield, L. (2003). *Clinical supervisor training: An interactive CD-ROM training program for the helping professions.* Boston: Allyn & Bacon.

Baptiste, S. (2005). Changing face of entry to occupational therapy practice: Some personal reflections for a person environment perspective. *Australian Occupational Therapy Journal, 52,* 179–180.

Benner, P. (1984). *From novice to expert: Excellence and power in clinical nursing practice.* Menlo Park, CA: Addison-Wesley.

Benner, P. (2004). Using the Dreyfus model of skill acquisition to describe and interpret skill acquisition and clinical judgment in nursing practice and education. *Bulletin of Science, Technology, and Society, 24,* 188–199.

Bennett, R. (2003). Clinical education: Perceived abilities/qualities of clinical educators and team supervision of students. *Physiotherapy, 89,* 432–440.

Bernard, J. M., & Goodyear, R. K. (2004). *Fundamentals of clinical supervision* (3rd ed.). Boston: Allyn & Bacon.

Blake, T. (2005). Journaling: An active learning technique. *International Journal of Nursing Scholarship, 2,* 1–13.

Blanchard, K., & Johnson, S. (1981). *The one minute manager.* New York: William Morrow.

Blanchard, K., & Zagarmi, P. (1985). *Leadership and the one minute manager: Increasing effectiveness through situational leadership.* New York: William Morrow.

Bloom, B. (1956). *Taxonomy of educational objectives, handbook 1: The cognitive domain.* New York: David McKay.

Boud, D. (2001). Using journal writing to enhance reflective practice. *New Directions for Adult and Continuing Education, 90,* 9–17.

Boud, D., Keogh, R., & Walker, D. (1985). *Reflection: Turning experience into learning.* London: Kogan Page.

Brackett, J. R. (1904). *Supervision and education in charity.* New York: Macmillan.

Bradley, L. J. (1989). *Counselor supervision: Principles, process, and practice.* Muncie, IN: Accelerated Development.

Brookfield, S. (1986). *Understanding and facilitating adult learning.* Buckingham, England: Open University Press.

Brookfield, S. (1987). *Developing critical thinkers: Challenging adults to explore alternative ways of thinking and acting.* San Francisco: Jossey-Bass.

Brown, T. (1998). The advantages of fieldwork in a community-based setting without occupational therapy: The supervisor's perspective. *Mental Health Special Interest Section Quarterly, 21*(2), 1–2.

Bruner, J. (1961). *The process of education.* Cambridge, MA: Harvard University Press.

Burns, E. M. (1965). *Encyclopedia of social work.* New York: National Association of Social Workers.

Campbell, J. (2000). *Becoming an effective supervisor: A workbook for counselors and psychotherapists.* Philadelphia: Taylor & Francis.

Campbell, J. M. (2006). *Essentials of clinical supervision.* Hoboken, NJ: Wiley.

Cara, E., & MacRae, A. (Eds.). (2005). *Psychosocial occupational therapy: A clinical practice* (2nd ed.). Clifton Park, NY: Thomson Delmar Learning.

Caspi, J., & Reid, W. (2002). *Educational supervision in social work: A task-centered model for field instruction and staff development.* New York: Columbia University Press.

Cermak, S. (1976). Community-based learning in occupational therapy. *American Journal of Occupational Therapy, 30,* 157–161.

Christie, A. (1999). A meaningful occupation: The just-right challenge. *Australian Journal of Occupational Therapy, 46,* 52–68.

Christie, B., Joyce, P., & Moeller, P. (1985). Fieldwork experience: Part II. The supervisor's dilemma. *American Journal of Occupational Therapy, 39,* 675–681.

Clouten, N., Homma, M., & Shimada, R. (2006). Clinical education and cultural diversity in physical therapy: Clinical performance of minority student physical therapists and the expectations of clinical instructors. *Physiotherapy Theory and Practice, 22,* 1–15.

Cohn, E., & Crist, P. (1995). Back to the future: New approaches to fieldwork education. *American Journal of Occupational Therapy, 49,* 103–106.

Cohn, E., Dooley, N., & Simmons, L. (2001). Collaborative learning applied to fieldwork education. *Occupational Therapy in Mental Health, 15,* 69–83.

Cohn, E., & Frum, D. (1988). Fieldwork supervision: More education is warranted. *American Journal of Occupational Therapy, 42,* 325–327.

Collins, G., Cassie, J., & Daggett, C. (1978). The role of the attending physician in clinical teaching. *Journal of Medical Education, 35,* 518–524.

Constantine, M., Warren, A., & Miville, M. (2005) White racial identity interactions in supervision: Implications for supervisees' multicultural counseling competence. *Journal of Consulting Psychology, 52,* 490–496.

Costa, D. (2004). *The essential guide to occupational therapy fieldwork education: Resources for today's educators and practitioners.* Bethesda, MD: AOTA Press.

Costa, D. (2007). The collaborative fieldwork model. *OT Practice, 12*(1), 25–26.

Covey, S. (1994). *First things first.* New York: Free Press.

Crepeau, E., & LaGarde, T. (1991). *Self-paced instruction for clinical education and supervision.* Rockville, MD: American Occupational Therapy Association.

Crist, P., Munoz, J., Hansen, A., Benson, J., & Provident, I. (2005). The practice–scholar program: An academic–practice partnership to promote the scholarship of "best practices." *Occupational Therapy in Health Care, 19*(1/2), 71–93.

Cross, V. (1995). Perceptions of the ideal clinical educator in physiotherapy education. *Physiotherapy, 81,* 506–513.

Cross, V. (1996). Introducing learning contracts into physiotherapy clinical education. *Physiotherapy, 82,* 21–27.

Cross, V., Moore, A., Morris, J., Caladine, L., Hilton, R., & Bristow, H. (2006). *The practice-based educator: A reflective tool for continuing professional development and accreditation.* Hoboken, NJ: Wiley.

Daloz, L. (1999). *Mentor: Guiding the journey of adult learners.* San Francisco: Jossey-Bass.

D'Andrea, M., Daniels, J., & Heck, R. (1991). Evaluating the impact of multicultural counseling training. *Journal of Counseling and Development, 70,* 143–150.

Dawson, J. B. (1926). The casework supervisor in a family agency. *Family, 6,* 293–295.

DeClute, J., & Ladyshewsky, R. (1993). Enhancing clinical competence: Using a collaborative clinical education model. *Physical Therapy, 73,* 683–688.

Dewey, J. (1933). *How we think: A restatement of the relation of reflective thinking to the educative process.* Boston: D. C. Heath.

Dewey, J. (1974). *John Dewey on education: Selected writings* (R. D. Archambeault, Ed.). Chicago: University of Chicago Press.

Dour, M., Grey, C., & Michaelsen, S. (2007). Collaborative learning: The student perspective. *OT Practice, 12*(4), 9–10.

Dreyfus, H., & Dreyfus, S. (1986). *Mind over machine: The power of human intuition and expertise in the era of the computer.* New York: Free Press.

Dunn, R. (2000). Learning styles: Theory, research, and practice. *National Forum of Applied Educational Research Journal, 13,* 3–22.

Dunn, R., & Dunn, K. (1998). *The complete guide to the learning styles inservice system.* Upper Saddle River, NJ: Prentice-Hall.

Early, M. (2000). *Mental health concepts and techniques for the occupational therapy assistant* (3rd ed.). Philadelphia: Lippincott.

Ekelman, B., Bello-Haas, V., Bazyk, J., & Bazyk, S. (2003). Developing cultural competence in occupational therapy and physical therapy education: A field immersion approach. *Journal of Allied Health, 32,* 131–137.

Ellis, M. (2001). Harmful supervision, a cause for alarm. *Journal of Counseling Psychology, 48,* 400–406.

Emery, M. (1984). Effectiveness of the clinical educator: Students' perspective. *Physical Therapy, 64,* 1079–1083.

Entwistle, N. (1987). A model of the teaching learning process. In J. Richardson, M. Eysenck, & W. Piper (Eds.), *Student learning* (pp. 13–28). Buckingham, England: Open University Press.

Falendar, C., & Shafranske, E. (2004). *Clinical supervision: A competency-based approach.* Washington, DC: American Psychological Association.

Fidler, G. (1966). Learning as a growth process: A conceptual framework for professional education. *American Journal of Occupational Therapy, 20,* 1–8.

Fish, D., & Twinn, S. (1997). *Quality clinical supervision in the healthcare professions: Principled approaches to practice.* Oxford, England: Butterworth-Heinemann.

Fish, D., Twinn, S., & Purr, B. (1991). Promoting reflection: The supervision of practice. In D. Fish, S. Twinn, & B. Purr (Eds.), *Health visiting and initial teacher training* (pp. 23–70). London: West London Institute Press.

Friedlander, M., Sigel, S., & Brenock, K. (1989). Parallel process in counseling and supervision: A case study. *Journal of Consulting Psychology, 36,* 149–157.

Frum, D., & Opacich, K. (1987). *Supervision: Development of therapeutic competence.* Rockville, MD: American Occupational Therapy Association.

Gabarini, J., & Pearlman, V. (1998). Fieldwork in home health care: A model for practice. *Education Special Interest Section Quarterly, 8*(4), 1–4.

Gagne, R. (1965). *The conditions of learning.* New York: Holt, Rineheart, & Winston.

Gandy, J. (2002). Preparation for teaching students in clinical settings. In K. Shepard, & G. Jensen (Eds.), *Handbook of teaching for physical therapists* (2nd ed., pp. 211–254). Woburn, MA: Butterworth-Heinemann.

Gilbert, M., & Evans, K. (2001). *Psychotherapy supervision: An integrative relational approach to psychotherapy supervision.* Philadelphia: Open University Press.

Graf, N., & Strebnicki, M. (2002). Using e-mail for clinical supervision in practicum: A qualitative analysis. *Journal of Rehabilitation, 68,* 1–15.

Grimm, T., & Massieon, M. (1998). Advantages of fieldwork in a community-based setting without occupational therapy: A student's perspective. *Mental Health Special Interest Section Quarterly, 21*(2), 2–4.

Grossman, J. (1974). Community experience for students. *American Journal of Occupational Therapy, 28,* 589–591.

Happell, B. (2004). Facilitating the professional development role of clinicians: Evaluating the impact of the clinician–trainer program. *Nurse Education in Practice, 4,* 83–90.

Harden, R., & Crosby, J. (2000). The good teacher is more than lecturer: The twelve roles of the teacher. *Medical Teacher, 22,* 334–347.

Hart, G. (1982). *The process of clinical education.* Baltimore: University Park Press.

Hawkins, P., & Shohet, R. (1989). *Supervision in the helping professions.* Buckingham, England: Open University Press.

Hawkins, P., & Shohet, R. (2000). *Supervision in the helping professions* (2nd ed.). Philadelphia: Open University Press.

Haynes, R., Corey, G., & Moulton, P. (2003). *Clinical supervision in the helping professions: A practical guide.* Pacific Grove, CA: Brooks/Cole–Thomson Learning.

Hays, P. (2001). *Addressing cultural complexities in practice: A framework for clinicians and counselors.* Washington, DC: American Psychological Association.

Helms, J. (1995). An update of Helms's White and people of color racial identity models. In J. G. Ponterotto, J. Casas, L. Susuki, & C. Alexander, (Eds.) *Handbook of multicultural counseling* (pp. 181–198). Thousand Oaks, CA: Sage.

Helms, J. (1999). Another meta-analysis of the White Racial Identity Scale. *Journal of Counseling Psychology, 44,* 13–16.

Hersey, P., Blanchard, K., & Johnson, D. (1996). *Management of organizational behavior: Utilizing human resources* (7th ed.). Upper Saddle River, NJ: Prentice-Hall.

Hersey, P., Blanchard, K., & Johnson, D. (2000). *Management of organizational behavior: Leading human resources* (8th ed.). Upper Saddle River, NJ: Prentice Hall.

Hesketh, E., Bagnall, G., Buckley, E. G., Friedman, M., Goodall, E., Harden, R., et al. (2001). A framework for developing excellence as a clinical educator. *Medical Education, 35,* 555–564.

Hesketh, E., & Laidlaw, J. (2002a). Developing the teaching instinct: 2. Supervision. *Medical Teacher, 24,* 364–367.

Hesketh, E., & Laidlaw, J. (2002b). Developing the teaching instinct: 3. Facilitating learning. *Medical Teacher, 24,* 479–482.

Hess, A. K. (Ed.). (1980). *Psychotherapy supervision: Theory, research, and practice.* New York: Wiley.

Hess, A. (1986). Growth in supervision: Stages of supervisee and supervisor development. *Clinical Supervisor, 41*(1–2), 51–67.

Higgs, J., & McAllister, L. (2005). The lived experiences of clinical educators with implications for their preparation, support, and professional development. *Learning in Health and Social Care, 4,* 156–171.

Hillerbrand, E. (1989). Cognitive differences between experts and novices: Implications for group supervision. *Journal of Counseling and Development, 67,* 293–296.

Hird, J., Cavalieri, C., Dulko, J., Felice, A., & Ho, T. (2001). Visions and realities: Supervisee perspective of multicultural supervision. *Journal of Multicultural Counseling and Development, 29,* 114–130.

Hoffman, M., Hill, C., Holmes, S., & Freitas, G. (2005). Supervisor perspectives on the process and outcome of giving easy, difficult, or no feedback to supervisees. *Journal of Counseling Psychology, 52,* 3–13.

Holloway, E. (1995). *Clinical supervision: A systems approach.* Thousand Oaks, CA: Sage.

Holly, M. (1997). *Keeping a professional journal.* Geelong, Australia: Deakin University Press.

Honey, P., & Mumford, A. (2000). *The learning styles questionnaire: 80 item version.* Berkshire, England: Peter Honey Publications.

Hook, A., & Lawson-Porter, A. (2003). The development and evaluation of a field-work educator's training programme for allied health professionals. *Medical Teacher, 25,* 527–536.

Hummell, J. (1997). Effective fieldwork supervision: Occupational therapy student perspectives. *Australian Occupational Therapy Journal, 44,* 147–157.

Irby, D. (1986). Clinical teaching and the clinical teacher. *Journal of Medical Education, 61*(9), 35–45.

Jantzen, A., & Yerxa, E. (1966). *The clinical experience.* Rockville, MD: American Occupational Therapy Association.

Johnson, D., & Johnson, R. (1991). *Learning together and alone: Cooperative, competitive, and individualistic learning.* Boston: Allyn & Bacon.

Jolly, B. (1999). Clinical logbooks: Recoding clinical experiences may not be enough. *Medical Education, 33,* 86–88.

Jung, C. (1969). *On the nature of the psyche* (R. E. C. Hull, Trans.). Princeton, NJ: Princeton University Press.

Jung, B., Sainsbury, S., Grum, R., Wilkins, S., & Tryssenaar, J. (2002). Collaborative fieldwork education with student occupational therapists and student occupational therapy assistants. *Canadian Journal of Occupational Therapy, 69,* 95–103.

Kadushin, A. (1976). *Supervision in social work.* New York: Columbia University Press.

Kadushin, A. (1992). *Supervision in social work* (3rd ed.). New York: Columbia University Press.

Kadushin, A. (2002*). Supervision in social work* (4th ed.). New York: Columbia University Press.

Kaslow, F. (1977). *Supervision, consultation, and staff training in the helping professions.* San Francisco: Jossey-Bass.

Kaufman, D. (2003). ABC of learning and teaching in medicine: Applying educational theory in practice. *British Medical Journal, 326,* 213–216.

Kautzmann, L. (1990). Clinical teaching: Fieldwork supervisors' attitudes and values. *American Journal of Occupational Therapy, 44,* 835–838.

Kearney, P. (2004). *The influence of competing paradigms in occupational therapy education: A brief history.* Retrieved December 2, 2005, from http:///www.newfoundations.com/History/OccTher.html

Keenan, M., Hoover, P., & Hoover, R. (1988). Leadership: Theory lets clinical instructors guide students toward autonomy. *Nursing Health Care, 9,* 82–86.

Kennedy-Jones, M. (2004). Contract learning. In M. Rose & D. Best (Eds.), *Transforming practice through clinical education, professional supervision, and mentoring* (pp. 249–257). New York: Elsevier.

Kilminster, S., & Jolly, B. (2000). Effective supervision in clinical practice settings: A literature review. *Medical Education, 43,* 827–840.

Kitzrow, M. (2001). A model of supervisory style based on psychological type. *Clinical Supervisor, 20,* 133–146.

Knowles, M. (1980a). *The modern practice of adult education: From pedagogy to androgogy.* New York: Cambridge University Press.

Knowles, M. (1980b). *The theory and practice of adult education.* Chicago: Follett.

Knowles, M. (1983). The modern practice of education: From pedagogy to andragogy. In M. Jobling & M. Tight (Eds.), *Adult learning and education*. London: Croom Helm.

Knowles, M., Holton, E., & Swanson, R. (2005). *The adult learner: The definitive classic in adult education and human resource development* (6th ed.). Burlington, MA: Elsevier.

Kolb, D. (1984). *Experiential learning: Experience as a source of learning and development*. Englewood Cliffs, NJ: Prentice Hall.

Kutzik, A. (1977a). The medical field. In F. Kaslow (Ed.), *Supervision, consultation, and staff training in the helping professions* (pp. 1–23). San Francisco: Jossey-Bass.

Ladany, N., & Melincoff, D. (1999). The nature of counselor supervisor nondisclosure. *Counselor Education and Supervision, 38,* 161–176.

Ladyshewsky, R. (1996a). Cross cultural clinical supervision: The impact of culture on teaching and learning. In *Different approaches: Theory and practice in higher education—Proceedings of the HERDSA Conference 1996*. Perth, Western Australia.

Ladyshewsky, R. (1996b). *Cross cultural clinical supervision/education: The SE Asian experience*. Retrieved November 18, 2005, from http://lsn.curtin.edu/tlf/tlfl 1996/ladyshewsky2.html

Lehrman-Waterman, D., & Ladany, N. (2001). Development and validity of the evaluation process within supervision inventory [Special Issue]. *Journal of Counseling Psychology, 48,* 15–24.

Loganbill, C., Hardy, E., & Delworth, U. (1982). Supervision: A conceptual model. *Counseling Psychologist, 10,* 3–42.

Loevinger, J. (1977). *Ego development: Conceptions and theories*. San Francisco, CA: Jossey-Bass.

Lopez, A., & Maggio, E. (2005, December). *Legal issues in fieldwork education: What every clinical instructor needs to know*. Workshop presented at the MOTEC [Metropolitan New York and New Jersey Occupational Therapy Education Council] Joint Clinical Council Day, New York.

MacKenzie, L., Zakrzewski, L., Walker, C., & McCluskey, A. (2001). Meeting the educational needs of fieldwork supervisors: A collaborative workshop developed by New South Wales occupational therapy fieldwork coordinators. *Australian Occupational Therapy Journal, 48,* 1–10.

Magnuson, S., Wilcoxon, S., & Norem, K. (2000). A profile of lousy supervision: Experienced counselors' perspectives. *Counselor Education and Supervision, 39,* 189–202.

Maslow, A. (1970). *Motivation and personality*. New York: Harper & Row.

Matheson, R. (2003). Promoting the integration of theory and practice by the use of a learning contract. *International Journal of Therapy and Rehabilitation, 10,* 264–270.

McAllister, L. (2000). Using adult education theories: Facilitating others' learning in professional practice settings. In S. Brown & S. Ryan (Eds.), *Becoming an advanced healthcare practitioner* (pp. 216–238). Philadelphia: Butterworth-Heinemann.

McAllister, L. (2001). *The experience of being a clinical educator*. Unpublished PhD thesis, University of Sydney, Australia.

McDonald, E. (1971). *The process of education and training in occupational therapy.* Presented at the 5th International Congress of the World Federation of Occupational Therapy, Zurich, Germany.

Merriam-Webster's New Collegiate Dictionary. (2003). Supervision (p. 1255). Springfield, MA: Merriam-Webster.

Meyer, L. (2000). Athletic training clinical instructors as situational leaders. *Journal of Athletic Training, 37*(4, Suppl.), S261–S265.

Mezirow, J. (1991). *Transformative dimensions of adult learning.* New York: Jossey-Bass.

Milan, F., Parish, S., & Reichgott, M. (2006). A model for educational feedback based on clinical communication skills strategies: Beyond the "feedback sandwich." *Teaching and Learning in Medicine, 18,* 42–47.

Milne, D., & James, I. (2002). The observed impact of training on competence in clinical supervision. *British Journal of Clinical Psychology, 41,* 55–72.

Nelson, M., & Friedlander, M. (2001). A close look at conflictual supervisory relationships: The trainee's perspective. *Journal of Counseling Psychology, 48,* 384–395.

Nilsson, J., & Anderson, M. (2004). Supervising international students: The role of acculturation, role ambiguity, and multicultural discussions. *Professional Psychology: Research and Practice, 35,* 306–312.

Opacich, K. (1995). Is an educational philosophy missing from the fieldwork solution? *American Journal of Occupational Therapy, 49,* 160–164.

Palmer, P. (1998). *The courage to teach: Exploring the inner landscape of a teacher's life.* San Francisco: Jossey-Bass.

Page, S., & Wosket, V. (1994). *Supervising the counselor: A cyclical model.* New York: Routledge.

Pavlov, I. P. (1927). *Conditioned reflexes: An investigation of the physiological activity of the cerebral cortex* (G. V. Anrep, Trans.). London: Oxford University Press.

Pederson, P. (2000). *A handbook for developing multicultural awareness* (3rd ed.). Alexandria, VA: American Counseling Association.

Perry, W. G. Jr. (1970). *Forms of intellectual and ethical development in the college years.* New York: Holt, Rinehart, & Winston.

Peters, J., & Armstrong, J. (1998). Collaborative learning: People laboring together to construct knowledge. *New Directions for Adult and Continuing Education, 79,* 75–85.

Piaget, J. (1970). *Science of education and the psychology of the child.* New York: Viking.

Plack, M., Driscoll, M., Blissett, S., McKenna, R., & Plack, T. (2005). A method for assessing reflective journal writing. *Journal of Allied Health, 34,* 199–208.

Ponterotto, J., Potere, J., & Johansen, A. (2002). The Quick Discrimination Index (QDI): Normative data and user guidelines for counseling researchers. *Journal of Multicultural Counseling and Development, 30,* 192–199.

Powell, D. (1993). *Clinical supervision in alcohol and drug abuse counseling: Principles, models, methods.* San Francisco: Jossey-Bass.

Privott, C. (1998). *The fieldwork anthology: A classic research and practice collection.* Bethesda, MD: American Occupational Therapy Association.

Prochaska, J. O., DiClemente, C. C., & Norcross, J. C. (1992). In search of how people change: Applications to addictive behaviors. *American Psychologist, 47,* 1102–1114.

Proctor, B. (1991). On being a trainer. In W. Dryden & B. Thorne (Eds.). *Training and supervision for counseling in action* (pp. 49–73). London: Sage.

Quiroga, V. (1995). *Occupational therapy: The first 30 years—1900 to 1930.* Bethesda, MD: American Occupational Therapy Association.

Robinson, V. (1936). *Supervision in social casework.* Chapel Hill: University of North Carolina Press.

Rodenhauser, P. (1994). Toward a multidimensional model for psychotherapy supervision based on developmental stages. *Journal of Psychotherapy Practice and Research, 3,* 1–15.

Rogers, C. (1969). *Freedom to learn.* Columbus, OH: Merrill.

Ronnestad, M., & Skovholt, T. (2003). The journey of the counselor and therapist: Research and findings and perspectives on professional development. *Journal of Career Development, 30,* 5–44.

Rose, M., & Best, D. (Eds.). (2005). *Transforming practice through clinical education, professional supervision, and mentoring.* Philadelphia: Elsevier.

Ryan, J. (1991). The function of student supervision. In American Occupational Therapy Association (Ed.), *Self-paced instruction for clinical education and supervision* (pp. 139–158). Rockville, MD: American Occupational Therapy Association

Scheidt, P., Lazoritz, S., Ebbeling, W. L., Figelman, A. R., Moessner, H. F., & Singer, J. E. (1986). Evaluation of a system providing feedback to students on video-taped patient encounters. *Journal of Medical Education, 61,* 585–590.

Schön, D. (1983). *The reflective practitioner: How professionals think in action.* New York: Basic Books.

Schön, D. (1987). *Educating the reflective practitioner.* San Francisco: Jossey-Bass.

Schwartz, K. (1984). An approach to the supervision of students on fieldwork. *American Journal of Occupational Therapy, 38,* 393–397.

Scott, S. (2000). Community-based fieldwork opportunities. *OT Practice, 5*(11), 14–18.

Shanfield, S., Hetherly, V., & Matthews, K. (2001). Excellent supervision: The residents' perspective. *Journal of Psychotherapy Practice and Research, 10,* 23–27.

Shorndike, A., & Howell, D. (2001). The reindeer of hope: An occupational therapy program in a homeless shelter. *Occupational Therapy in Health Care, 15*(1/2), 57–68.

Skinner, B. F. (1954). The science of learning and the art of teaching. *Harvard Educational Review, 24,* 86–97.

Stillman, P., Sabers, D., & Redfield, B. (1976). The use of paraprofessionals to teach interviewing skills. *Pediatrics, 58,* 165–169.

Stoltenberg, C., McNeill, B., & Delworth, U. (1998). *IDM: An integrated developmental model for supervising counselors and therapists.* San Francisco: Jossey-Bass.

Strohschein, J., Hagler, P., & May, L. (2002). Assessing the need for change in clinical education practices. *Physical Therapy, 82,* 160–172.

Suarez-Balcazar, Y., Hammel, J., Helfrich, C., Thomas, J., Wilson, T., & Head-Ball, D. (2005). A model of university–community partnerships for occupational therapy scholarship and practice. *Occupational Therapy in Health Care, 19*(1/2), 47–70.

Sue, D., Arredondo, P., & McDavis, R. (1992). Multicultural counseling competencies and standards: A call to the profession. *Journal of Counseling and Development, 70,* 477–486.

Sullivan, T., & Finlayson, M. (2000). Role-emerging fieldwork at the University of Manitoba. *Occupational Therapy Now, 2*(3), 13–14, 24.

Sweeney, G., Webley, P., & Treacher, A. (2001a). Supervision in occupational therapy: Part 1. The supervisor's anxieties. *British Journal of Occupational Therapy, 64*, 337–345.

Sweeney, G., Webley, P., & Treacher, A. (2001b). Supervision in occupational therapy: Part 2. Accommodating the supervisor and the supervisee. *British Journal of Occupational Therapy, 64*, 426–431.

Titchen, A., & Higgs, J. (2001). A dynamic framework for the enhancement of health professional practice in an uncertain world: The practice–knowledge interface. In J. Higgs & A. Titchen (Eds.), *Practice knowledge and expertise* (pp. 215–225). Oxford: Butterworth-Heinemann.

Tummal-Narra, P. (2004). Dynamics of race and culture in the supervisory encounter. *Psychoanalytic Psychology, 21*, 300–311.

van der Hem-Stokroos, H., Daelmans, H., van der Vleuten, C., Haarman, H., & Scherpbier, A. (2003). A qualitative study of constructive clinical learning experiences. *Medical Teacher, 25*, 120–126.

van Ooijen, E. (2000). *Clinical supervision: A practical guide.* London: Churchill-Livingstone.

Vendrely, A., & Carter, R. (2004). The influence of training on the rating of physical therapist student performance in the clinical setting. *Journal of Allied Health, 33*, 62–69.

Vygotsky, L. S. (1962). *Thought and language.* Cambridge, MA: MIT Press.

Vygotsky, L. S. (1978). *Mind in society.* Cambridge, MA: Harvard University Press.

Wales, C., Nardi, A., & Stager, R. (1993). Emphasizing critical thinking and problem-solving. In L. Curry, J. F. Wergin, & Associates. (Eds.), *Educating professionals: Responding to new expectations for competence and accountability* (pp. 178–226). San Francisco: Jossey-Bass.

Watkins, C. (1990). Development of the psychotherapy supervisor. *Psychotherapy, 27*, 553–560.

Westberg, J., & Jason, H. (1993). *Collaborative clinical education: The foundation for effective health care.* New York: Springer.

Westberg, J., & Jason, H. (2001). *Fostering reflection and providing feedback: Helping others learn from experience.* New York: Springer.

Whiffen, R. (1982). The use of videotape in supervision. In R. Whiffin & J. Byng-Hall, J. (Eds.), *Family therapy supervision: Recent developments in practice.* New York: Academic Press.

Whitcomb, B. (1951). Methods of clinical instruction in physical therapy. *Physical Therapy, 31*, 129–134.

Whitcombe, S. (2001). Using learning contracts in fieldwork education: The views of occupational therapy students and those responsible for their supervision. *British Journal of Occupational Therapy, 64*, 552–558.

White, E. B. (1952). *Charlotte's web.* New York: HarperCollins.

Wickham, J. (2005a, March 17). Approaches to learning. *Therapy Weekly*, pp. 11–13.

World Health Organization. (2001). *International classification of functioning, disability, and health (ICF).* Retrieved March 30, 2007, from www.who.int/classifications/icf/en/.

Yerxa, E. J. (1984). Duties and responsibilities of fieldwork educators in the educational process. In American Occupational Therapy Association (Ed.), *Guide to fieldwork education* (pp. 161–168). Rockville, MD: American Occupational Therapy Association.

Zea, M., Asner-Self, K., Birman, D., & Buki, L. (2003). The abbreviated multidimensional acculturation scale: Empirical validation with two Latino/Latina samples. *Cultural Diversity and Ethnic Minority Psychology, 9,* 107–126.

Recommended Reading (see also Annotated Bibliography)

Aiken, F., Menaker, L., & Barsky, L. (2001). Fieldwork education: The future of occupational therapy depends on it. *Occupational Therapy International, 8*(2), 86–95.

Aten, J., & Hernandez, B. (2004). Addressing religion in clinical supervision: A model. *Psychotherapy: Theory, Research, Practice, Training, 41,* 152–160.

Bailey, C. (2004). Reflecting on supervision training courses—The heart of the matter. *Counselling and Psychotherapy Journal, 15*(10), 36–39.

Baker, S., Exum, H., & Tyler, R. (2002). The developmental process of clinical supervisors in training: An investigation of the supervisor complexity model. *Counselor Education and Supervision, 42*(1), 15–30.

Barkley, E., Cross, P., & Major, C. (2004). *Collaborative learning techniques: A handbook for college faculty.* Somerset, NJ: Jossey-Bass.

Barrett, K. (2000). The time is now for innovative fieldwork sites and practice. *Education Special Interest Section Quarterly, 10*(2), 1–2.

Boniface, G. (2002). Understanding reflective practice in occupational therapy. *British Journal of Therapy and Rehabilitation, 9,* 292–298.

Bossers, A., Cook, J., Polatajko, H., & Lane, C. (1997). Understanding the role-emerging fieldwork placement. *Canadian Journal of Occupational Therapy, 64*(2), 70–81.

Boyd, M., & Gabarini, J. (2001). Helping build healthy communities through OT fieldwork. *OT Practice, 6*(10), 17–21.

Boyle, J., Sammon, S., Montemuro, M., Blythe, J., & Morrison, F. (1998). Preparing clinical educators: Interdisciplinary collaboration. *Gerontology and Geriatrics Education, 19*(2), 31–45.

Brown, G., Esdaile, S., & Ryan, S. (2003). *Becoming an advanced healthcare practitioner.* New York: Butterworth-Heinemann.

Brownstein, L., Rettie, C., & George, C. (1998). A programme to prepare instructors for clinical teaching. *Perfusion, 13,* 59–65.

Cara, E. (2005). Fieldwork supervision in mental health settings. In E. Cara & A. MacRae (Eds.), *Psychosocial occupational therapy: A clinical practice* (2nd ed.). Clifton Park, NY: Thomson Delmar Learning.

Clouder, L., & Sellars, J. (2004). Reflective practice and clinical supervision: An interprofessional perspective. *Journal of Advanced Nursing, 46,* 262–269.

Cockrell, K., Caplow, J., & Donaldson, J. (2000). A context for learning: Collaborative groups in the problem-based learning environment. *Review of Higher Education, 23,* 347–363.

Cole, M. (2005). Reflection in healthcare practice: Why is it useful and how might it be done? *Work Based Learning in Primary Care, 3,* 13–22.

Cottrell, D., Kilminster, S., Jolly, B., & Grant, J. (2002). What is effective supervision and how does it happen? A critical incident study. *Medical Education, 36,* 1042–1049.

Davis, J. (2006). The importance of the community of practice in identity development. *Internet Journal of Allied Health Sciences and Practice, 4*(3), 1–8.

Dewey, J. (1938). *Experience and education.* New York: Collier Books.

Donohue, M. (2001). Group leadership by occupational therapy students in community centers: Learning transitional roles. *Occupational Therapy in Health Care, 15*(1/2), 85–98.

Doubt, L., Paterson, M., & O'Riordan, A. (2004). Clinical education in private practice. *Journal of Allied Health, 33,* 47–50.

Douglas, K., Hosokawa, M., & Lawler, F. (1988). *A practical guide to clinical teaching in medicine.* New York: Springer.

Dye, D., & Bender, D. (2006). Duty and liability surrounding clinical internships: What every internship coordinator should know. *Journal of Allied Health, 35,* 169–173.

Edwards, D., Cooper, L., Burnard, P., Hannigan, B., Juggesur, T., Adams, J., et al. (2005). Factors influencing the effectiveness of clinical supervision. *Journal of Psychiatric and Mental Health Nursing, 12,* 405–414.

Fall, M., & Sutton, J. (2004). *Clinical supervision: A handbook for practitioners.* Boston: Pearson Education.

Fisher, A., & Savin-Baden, M. (2002). Modernizing fieldwork: Part 2. Realizing the new agenda. *British Journal of Occupational Therapy, 65,* 275–282.

Forneris, S., & Peden-McAlpine, C. (2006). Contextual learning: A reflective learning intervention for nursing education. *International Journal of Nursing Education Scholarship, 3,* 1–17.

Friedland, J., Polatajko, H., & Gage, M. (2001). Expanding the boundaries of occupational therapy practice through fieldwork experiences: Descriptions of a provincially funded community development project. *Canadian Journal of Occupational Therapy, 68,* 301–309.

Guyer, J., Odom, C., & Gandy, J. (2003). History of clinical education in physical therapy in the United States. *Journal of Physical Therapy Education, 17*(3), 34–43.

Hauer, P., Straub, C., & Wolf, S. (2005). Learning styles of allied health students using Kolb's LSI-Iia. *Journal of Allied Health, 34,* 177–182.

Hayward, K., Kochniuk, L., Powell, L., & Peterson, T. (2005). Changes in students' perceptions of interdisciplinary practice reaching the older adult through mobile service delivery. *Journal of Allied Health, 34,* 192–198.

Hentz, P., & Lauterbach, S. (2005). Becoming self-reflective: Caring for self and others. *International Journal for Human Caring, 9,* 24–28.

Higgs, J., & Edward, H. (Eds.). (1999). *Educating beginning practitioners: Challenges for health professional education.* Woburn, MA: Butterworth-Heinemann.

Holmes, W. (2006). Occupational therapy students and emerging practice: A pilot study. *Journal of Allied Health, 35,* e204–e214.

Hubbard, S. (2000). A case example of remote supervision. *OT Practice, 5*(24), 16–18.

Inspiring future generations of occupational therapists [Editorial]. (2005). *Australian Occupational Therapy Journal, 52,* 269–270.

Jones, A. (1998). Getting going with clinical supervision: An introductory seminar. *Journal of Advanced Nursing, 27,* 560–566.

Kember, D. (Ed.). (2001). *Reflective teaching and learning in the health professions: Action research in professional education.* Oxford, England: Blackwell.

Kessler, P., & Lund, C. (2004). Reflective journaling: Developing an online journal for distance education. *Nurse Educator, 29,* 20–24.

Kinsella, E. (2001). Examining your philosophy of practice: A reflective approach to professional development. *Occupational Therapy Now, 3,* 10–12.

Laidley, T., & Braddock, C. (2000). Role of adult learning theory in evaluating and designing strategies for teaching residents in ambulatory settings. *Advances in Health Sciences Education, 5,* 43–54.

Langlois, J., & Thach, S. (2001, May). Teaching and learning styles in the clinical setting. *Family Medicine, 33,* 344–346.

Launer, J. (2005). Reflective practice and clinical supervision: Teaching supervision in small groups. *Work Based Learning in Primary Care, 3,* 263–266.

Launer, J. (2006). Reflective practice and clinical supervision: Emotion and interpretation in supervision. *Work Based Learning in Primary Care, 4,* 171–173.

Lyons, M., & Ziviani, J. (1995). Stereotypes, stigma, and mental illness: Learning from fieldwork experiences. *American Journal of Occupational Therapy, 49,* 1002–1008.

Martin, M., Morris, J., Moore, A., Sadlo, G., & Crouch, V. (2004). Evaluating practice education models in occupational therapy: Comparing 1:1, 2:1, and 3:1 placements. *British Journal of Occupational Therapy, 67,* 192–200.

McDonough, J., & Osterbrink, J. (2005). Learning styles: An issue in clinical education? *American Association of Nursing Anesthesia Journal, 73*(2), 89–93.

Merriam, S. (2001). Androgogy and self-directed learning: Pillars of adult learning theory. *New Directions for Adult and Continuing Education, 89,* 3–13.

Moore, A., Hilton, R., Morris, J., Caladine, L., & Bristow, H. (1997). *The clinical educator—Role development: A self-directed learning text.* New York: Churchill-Livingstone.

Packer, T., Paterson, M., Krupa, T., Avtchoukhova, L., Tchebotareva, L., & Krasnova, L. (2000). Client outcomes after student community fieldwork in Russia. *Occupational Therapy International, 7,* 191–197.

Palmer, P. (1998). *The courage to teach: Exploring the inner landscape of a teacher's life.* San Francisco: Jossey-Bass.

Patterson, M., Wilcox, S., & Higgs, J. (2006). Exploring dimensions of artistry in reflective practice. *Reflective Practice, 7,* 455–468.

Puliyel, M., Puliyel, J., & Puliyel, U. (1999). Drawing on adult learning theory to teach personal and professional values. *Medical Teacher, 21,* 513–515.

Reed, J., & Koliba, C. (1995). *Facilitating reflection: A manual for leaders and educators.* Retrieved May 13, 2003, from www.uvm.edu/~dewey/reflection_manual/index.html

Royle, J., Sammon, S., Montemuro, M., Blythe, J., & Morrison, F. (1998). Preparing clinical educators: Interdisciplinary collaboration. *Gerontology and Geriatrics Education, 19*(2), 31–45.

Sandars, J. (2006). Transformative learning: The challenge for reflective practice. *Work Based Learning in Primary Care, 4,* 6–10.

Shepard, K., & Jensen, G. (2002). *Handbook of teaching for physical therapist* (2nd ed.). Philadelphia: Butterworth-Heinemann.

Sloggett, K., Kim, N., & Cameron, D. (2003). Private practice: Benefits, barriers, and strategies of providing fieldwork placements. *Canadian Journal of Occupational Therapy, 70*(1), 42–50.

Smith, A., & Jack, K. (2005). Reflective practice: A meaningful task for students. *Nursing Standard, 19*(26), 33–37.

Stafford, E. (1986). Relationship between occupational therapy student learning styles and clinic performance. *American Journal of Occupational Therapy, 40,* 34–39.

Steele-Smith, S., & Armstrong, M. (2001). I would take more students but . . . : Student supervision strategies. *British Journal of Occupational Therapy, 64,* 549–551.

Stern, K. (2005). Academic–clinician partnerships: A model for outcomes research. *Occupational Therapy in Health Care, 19*(1/2), 95–106.

Storr, C., & Thomas, A. (2001). New techno-teaching tools: Do they have a place in clinical education? *Occupational Therapy Now, 3*(2), 7–9.

Su, W., Osisek, P., & Starnes, B. (2004). Applying the revised Bloom's taxonomy to a medical–surgical nursing lesson. *Nursing Educator, 29,* 116–120.

Su, W., Osisek, P., & Starnes, B. (2005). Using the revised Bloom's taxonomy in the clinical laboratory: Thinking skills involved in clinical reasoning. *Nurse Educator, 30,* 117–122.

Swedlove, F. (2006). Expanding horizons for occupational therapy students through fieldwork placements. *Occupational Therapy Now, 8*(5), 22–24.

Taylor, R., Fisher, G., & Kielhofner, G. (2005). Synthesizing research, education, and practice according to the scholarship of practice model: Two faculty models. *Occupational Therapy in Health Care, 19*(1/2), 107–122.

Thibeault, R. (2006). Globalisation, universities, and the future of occupational therapy: Dispatches for the majority world. *Australian Occupational Therapy Journal, 53,* 159–165.

Thomas, A., & Storr, C. (2005). WebCT in occupational therapy clinical education: Implementing and evaluating a tool for peer learning and interaction. *Occupational Therapy International, 12,* 162–179.

Totten, C., & Preatt, J. (2001). Innovation in fieldwork education: Working with the homeless population in Glasgow. *British Journal of Occupational Therapy, 64,* 559–563.

Wickham, J. (2005b, April 14). Using reflective practice as a learning tool in clinical supervision. *Therapy Weekly,* pp. 13–16.

Wilkins, S., & Jung, B. (2001). Establishing research, fieldwork, and service partnerships. *Physical and Occupational Therapy in Geriatrics, 19,* 65–78.

Williams, R., Sundelin, G., Foster-Sargeant, E., & Norman, G. (2000). Assessing the reliability of grading reflective journal writing. *Journal of Physical Therapy Education, 14*(2).

Wimpenny, K., Forsyth, K., Jones, C., Evans, E., & Colley, J. (2006). Group reflective supervision: Thinking with theory to develop practice. *British Journal of Occupational Therapy, 69,* 423–428.

Wood, J., Miller, T., & Hargrove, D. (2005). Clinical supervision in rural settings: A telehealth model. *Professional Psychology: Research and Practice, 36,* 173–179.

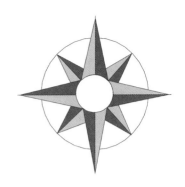

Appendix A.
Role Competencies for a
Fieldwork Educator

Purpose

These role competencies have been developed to assist educational programs in determining and/or evaluating the typical responsibilities of a fieldwork educator associated with an occupational therapy program. The competencies are based on the American Occupational Therapy Association's *Standards for Continuing Competence*. These role competencies are statements describing the typical values, knowledge, skills, and responsibilities that are needed to be successful in the role of a fieldwork educator. The competencies are general statements, as specific competencies may not apply to all situations. Each competency may be modified and should be considered a guideline for institutions or educational settings.

Standard 1. Knowledge

Occupational therapy practitioners shall demonstrate understanding and comprehension of the information required for the multiple roles they assume. In addition to the recognized competencies for occupational therapy practitioners, the fieldwork educator must be able to

- Facilitate the development of competent entry-level occupational therapy practitioners through the provision of supervised quality fieldwork experiences
- Develop learning activities and assignments that encompass the breadth and depth of knowledge in the profession and reinforce knowledge and skills leading to entry-level competency
- Demonstrate knowledge of effective learning processes that identify individual learning styles and use appropriate and individualized techniques for students at their fieldwork education site
- Demonstrate accurate and current knowledge of the contractual agreement between the colleges/universities and the fieldwork site
- Demonstrate the competence to develop and maintain proficiency in occupational therapy processes and supervision skills through investigation, formal education, continuing education, or self-study

- Maintain current knowledge of standards, rules, and regulations regarding supervision of students set by the state, accreditation bodies, and the fieldwork institution.

Standard 2. Critical Reasoning

Occupational therapy practitioners shall employ reasoning processes to make sound judgments and decisions within the context of their roles. In addition to the recognized competencies for occupational therapy practitioners, a fieldwork educator must be able to

- Effectively evaluate and share knowledge in the form of new materials, literature, and educational materials relating to fieldwork that enhance the lifelong learning of future occupational therapy practitioners
- Critically integrate and apply theory, literature, and research into practice at the fieldwork education site
- Critically evaluate the curriculum, particularly in terms of its components and their relationship to fieldwork education, and participate in curriculum development in relation to the best practice in the fieldwork setting
- Evaluate interpersonal dynamics among occupational therapy practitioners, other clinical and non-clinical personnel, clients, and students to resolve issues and determine action plans, including contacting the academic fieldwork coordinator
- Demonstrate the ability to communicate critical reasoning behind clinical practice decisions to students and encourage development of critical reasoning in the fieldwork student.

Standard 3. Interpersonal Skills

Occupational therapy practitioners shall develop and maintain their professional relationships with others within the context of their roles. In addition to the recognized competencies for occupational therapy practitioners, a fieldwork educator must be able to

- Project a positive image of the fieldwork program to the college or university, student, and community
- Demonstrate a competent and positive attitude towards practice and supervision that will result in effective development and mentoring of fieldwork students
- Effectively supervise and advise fieldwork students in relation to fieldwork and practice issues
- Effectively mediate interpersonal issues among students, clients, and staff
- Demonstrate positive, culturally sensitive interactions with diverse faculty, students, fieldwork coordinators, and practitioners

- Identify and clearly communicate both strengths and areas for improvement to students in a manner that encourages student growth as a practitioner.

Standard 4. Performance Skills

Occupational therapy practitioners shall demonstrate the expertise, attitudes, proficiencies, and ability to competently fulfill their roles. In addition to the recognized competencies for occupational therapy practitioners, a fieldwork educator must be able to

- Plan fieldwork experiences within his or her setting that will prepare ethical and competent practitioners
- Develop fieldwork course objectives, course materials, and educational activities and experiences that promote optimal learning for students
- Evaluate students' performance and learning outcomes in relation to fieldwork objectives of the program and the organization
- Design and implement a plan that develops and maintains accurate documentation of student performance, collaboration with academic curriculum, the fieldwork academic coordinator, and/or other documentation required for fieldwork experiences.

Standard 5. Ethical Reasoning

Occupational therapy practitioners shall identify, analyze, and clarify ethical issues or dilemmas in order to make responsible decisions within the changing context of their roles. In addition to the recognized competencies for occupational therapy practitioners, a fieldwork educator must be able to

- Act as a role model as an occupational therapy advocate and change agent in situations with professional, culturally competent, and ethical behavior
- Clarify and analyze fieldwork issues within an ethical framework for positive resolution.

Prepared by

Anne E. Dickerson, PhD, OTR/L, FAOTA,
   Professional Program Director/Chairperson PRODEC, Commission on Education

for

The Commission on Education
Linda Fazio, PhD, OTR/L, FAOTA, *Chairperson*

Adopted by the Representative Assembly 2005M284

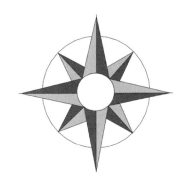

Appendix B.
Role Competencies for an
Academic Fieldwork Coordinator

Purpose

The development of these role competencies is to assist academic settings in determining and/or evaluating the typical responsibilities for an academic fieldwork coordinator in an occupational therapy or occupational therapy assistant educational program. The competencies are based on the American Occupational Therapy Association's *Standards for Continuing Competence.* These role competencies are statements describing the typical values, knowledge, skills, and responsibilities that are needed to be successful in this role. The competencies are general statements, and specific competencies may not apply to all situations. Each competency may be modified and should be considered guidelines for institutions.

Standard 1. Knowledge

Occupational therapy practitioners shall demonstrate understanding and comprehension of the information required for the multiple roles they assume. In addition to the recognized competencies for occupational therapy practitioners, an academic fieldwork coordinator must

- Demonstrate the expertise to be able to facilitate the development of future leaders in occupational therapy through student development in supervised quality fieldwork settings
- Develop a plan to continue competency in the breadth and depth of knowledge in the profession to incorporate into student learning
- Develop a plan to promote effective learning processes for students in the program and associated fieldwork education sites
- Demonstrate the competence to develop and maintain accurate and current knowledge of reimbursement issues, federal regulations concerning student services, legal issues concerning fieldwork experiences, and pertinent federal/state regulations such as the Americans With Disabilities Act
- Demonstrate the competence to develop and maintain accurate and current knowledge in contractual agreements between colleges/universities and fieldwork sites

- Demonstrate the competence to develop and maintain proficiency in fieldwork coordination skills through investigation, formal education, continuing education, or self-study.

Standard 2. Critical Reasoning

Occupational therapy practitioners shall employ reasoning processes to make sound judgments and decisions within the context of their roles. In addition to the recognized competencies for occupational therapy practitioners, an academic fieldwork coordinator must

- Facilitate professional development in teaching/fieldwork coordination through continuing education, research, or self-investigation
- Demonstrate the ability to effectively judge new materials, literature, and educational materials relating to fieldwork that enhance the lifelong learning of future occupational therapy practitioners
- Demonstrate the ability to critically integrate practice, theory, literature, and research in relation to practice in fieldwork education sites
- Demonstrate the ability to critically evaluate the curriculum, particularly in terms of fieldwork education, for participation in curriculum development
- Demonstrate the ability to evaluate interpersonal dynamics between occupational therapy practitioners and students to resolve issues and determine action plans.

Standard 3. Interpersonal Skills

Occupational therapy practitioners shall develop and maintain their professional relationships with others within the context of their roles. In addition to the recognized competencies for occupational therapy practitioners, an academic fieldwork coordinator must

- Project a positive image of the program both internally (within the college or university) and externally (within the community)
- Demonstrate a competent and positive attitude that will result in the development and mentoring of fieldwork educators
- Effectively mentor and advise students in relation to fieldwork education issues
- Effectively mediate interpersonal issues between students and fieldwork educators
- Demonstrate positive interactions with diverse faculty, students, fieldwork educators, and practitioners
- Demonstrate positive interactions with appropriate administrators and attorneys to facilitate contract negotiations.

Standard 4. Performance Skills

Occupational therapy practitioners shall demonstrate the expertise, attitudes, proficiencies, and ability to competently fulfill their roles. In addition to the recognized competencies for occupational therapy practitioners, an academic fieldwork coordinator must

- Demonstrate the ability to plan fieldwork experiences that will prepare ethical and competent practitioners for both traditional and emerging practice settings
- Demonstrate the expertise to develop fieldwork course objectives, course materials, and educational experiences that promote optimal learning for students
- Demonstrate the expertise to evaluate students' learning outcomes for fieldwork to meet the objectives of the program and the organization
- Demonstrate the ability to develop and implement a plan that effectively evaluates fieldwork educators and fieldwork sites to meet the objectives of the program and the organization
- Demonstrate the expertise to prepare, develop, and/or coordinate the legal contracts and associated issues for fieldwork establishment and maintenance
- Demonstrate the ability to design and implement a logical and justified system of fieldwork assignment for students and fieldwork educators
- Demonstrate the ability to plan and implement a plan that develops and maintains accurate documentation of student performance, collaboration with fieldwork settings and supervisors, and/or other documentation required for fieldwork experiences.

Standard 5. Ethical Reasoning

Occupational therapy practitioners shall identify, analyze, and clarify ethical issues or dilemmas in order to make responsible decisions within the changing context of their roles. In addition to the recognized competencies for occupational therapy practitioners, an academic fieldwork coordinator must

- Act as a role model as an occupational therapy advocate and change agent with professional and ethical behavior
- Clarify and analyze fieldwork issues within an ethical framework for positive resolution
- Identify and represent the educational and fieldwork settings accurately to ensure that legal contracts are appropriately documented.

Prepared by

Anne E. Dickerson, PhD, OTR/L, FAOTA,
Professional Program Director/Chairperson PRODEC, Commission on Education

for

The Commission on Education
Charlotte Brasic Royeen, PhD, OTR, FAOTA, *Chairperson*

Adopted by the Representative Assembly 2003M169

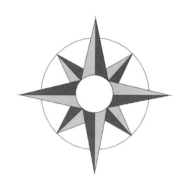

Appendix C.
Fieldwork Experience
Assessment Tool (FEAT)

Student's name:	Supervisor(s) names:		
Facility name:			
Fieldwork experience type (setting, population, level):		Date:	Week #:

Context

The Fieldwork Experience Assessment Tool (FEAT) is the result of an American Occupational Therapy Foundation qualitative study completed by six occupational therapy programs across the United States and Puerto Rico. Data were collected from fieldwork students and fieldwork educators. In their interviews, students and fieldwork educators described fieldwork education in terms of a dynamic triad of interaction among the environment, the fieldwork educator, and the student. Interviewees indicated that a positive educational experience occurred when a balance existed among these three key components.

Purpose

The FEAT identifies essential characteristics for each of the three key components. By providing a framework to explore the fieldwork experience, the FEAT can help students and fieldwork educators consider how to promote the best possible learning experience.

The purpose of the FEAT is to contribute to student and fieldwork educator discussions, so that reflection and problem solving can occur to enhance the fieldwork experience. The tool is designed to both assess the balance of the three key components and to facilitate discussion about student and fieldwork educator behaviors and attitudes and about environmental resources and challenges. By mutually identifying issues present during fieldwork, the fieldwork educator and student can use the FEAT as a tool to promote dialogue and foster the identification of strategies to facilitate the just-right challenge. The FEAT may be used early in fieldwork as a tool to promote dialogue or at anytime throughout fieldwork as the need for problem solving emerges.

Directions

In the Assessment Section, the FEAT is organized according to the three key components: **environment, fieldwork educator,** and **fieldwork student.** Under each component, essential characteristics and examples are listed. These examples are not all inclusive, and new descriptors may be added to individualize the tool for different settings. The fieldwork educator and student, either individually or together, should complete the FEAT by describing each component using the continuum provided at the top of each section (limited → just-right challenge → excessive).

Following the assessment portion of the FEAT, questions are provided to guide student and fieldwork educator discussion and problem solving. Collaboratively reflect upon the student and fieldwork educator descriptions on the FEAT to identify commonalities and differences between the two perspectives, and identify patterns across the key components. Based on these discussions, develop strategies for a more balanced fieldwork experience. Consider environmental experiences

A. Assessment Section

ENVIRONMENT	
I. VARIETY OF EXPERIENCES	**Descriptions** (Limited ⟷ Just-right challenge ⟷ Excessive)
A. Patients/Clients/Diagnoses - Different diagnoses - Range of abilities for given diagnosis (complexity, function–dysfunction) - Diversity of clients, including socio-economic and lifestyle	
B. Therapy Approaches - Engage in the entire therapy process (evaluation, planning, intervention, documentation) - Learn about different roles of therapist (direct service, consultation, education, and administration) - Use variety of activities with clients - Observe and use different frames of reference/theoretical approaches - Use occupation vs. exercise	
C. Setting Characteristics - Pace (setting demands, caseload quantity) - Delivery system	
II. RESOURCES	**Descriptions** (Limited ⟷ Just-right challenge ⟷ Excessive)
A. OT Staff - See others' strengths and styles - Have multiple role models, resources, and support	
B. Professional Staff - Observe and hear a different perspective on clients - See/experience cotreatments and teamwork to get whole-person perspective - Have others to share ideas and frustrations	
C. OT Students - Able to compare observations and experiences - Exchange ideas	

(Continued)

FIELDWORK EDUCATOR	
I. ATTITUDE	**Descriptions** (Limited ⟷ Just-right challenge ⟷ Excessive)
A. Likes Teaching/Supervising Students - Devotes time, invests in students - Enjoys mental workout, student enthusiasm	
B. Available/Accessible - Takes time	
C. Supportive - Patient - Positive and caring - Encourages questions - Encourages development of individual style	
D. Open - Accepting - Alternative methods - To student requests - Communication	
E. Mutual Respect	
II. TEACHING STRATEGIES	**Descriptions** (Limited ⟷ Just-right challenge ⟷ Excessive)
A. Structure - Organize information (set learning objectives, regular meetings) - Introduce treatment (dialogue, observation, treatment, dialogue) - Base structure on student need - Identify strategies for adjusting to treatment environment	
B. Graded Learning - Expose to practice (observe, model) - Challenge student gradually (reduce direction, probing questions, independence) - Base approach on student learning style - Individualize based on student's needs - Promote independence (trial and error)	

FIELDWORK EDUCATOR (*continued*)	
I. ATTITUDE	**Descriptions** (Limited ⟵⟶ Just-right challenge ⟵⟶ Excessive)
C. Feedback/Processing - Timely, confirming - Positive and constructive (balance) - Guide thinking - Promote clinical reasoning	
D. Teaching - Share resources and knowledge	
E. Team Skills - Include student as part of team	
F. Open - Accepting - Alternative methods - To student requests - Communication	
III. PROFESSIONAL ATTRIBUTES	**Descriptions** (Limited ⟵⟶ Just-right challenge ⟵⟶ Excessive)
A. Role Model - Sets good example - Enthusiasm for OT - Real person - Lifelong learning	
B. Teacher - Able to share resources and knowledge	
FIELDWORK STUDENT	
I. ATTITUDE	**Descriptions** (Limited ⟵⟶ Just-right challenge ⟵⟶ Excessive)
A. Responsible for Learning - Active learner (ask questions, consult) - Prepare (review, read, and research materials) - Self-direct (shows initiative, is assertive) - Learns from mistakes (self-corrects and grows)	

(Continued)

FIELDWORK STUDENT (*continued*)	
I. ATTITUDE	**Descriptions** (Limited ⟷ Just-right challenge ⟷ Excessive)

B. Open/Flexible
  - Sensitive to diversity (nonjudgmental)
  - Responsive to client/consumer needs
  - Flexible in thinking (makes adjustments, tries alternate approaches)	

C. Confident
  - Comfort in knowledge and abilities
  - Comfort with making and learning from mistakes (takes risks, branch out)
  - Comfort with independent practice (takes responsibility)
  - Comfort in receiving feedback	

D. Responsive to Supervision
  - Receptive to feedback (open-minded, accepts criticism)
  - Open communication (two-way)	

II. LEARNING BEHAVIORS	**Descriptions** (Limited ⟷ Just-right challenge ⟷ Excessive)

A. Independent
  - Has and uses knowledge and skills
  - Assumes responsibility of OT without needing direction
  - Incorporates feedback into behavioral changes
  - Uses "down time" productively
  - Becomes part of team	

B. Reflection
  - Self (processes feelings, actions, and feedback)
  - With others (supervisor, peers, others)	

C. Active in Supervision
  - Communicates needs to supervisor (seeks supervision for guidance and processing; expresses needs)
  - Asks questions	

B. Discussion Section: Questions to Facilitate Dialogue and Problem Solving

1. A positive fieldwork experience includes a balance between the environment, fieldwork educator, and student components. Collaboratively reflect upon the descriptions outlined by the student and fieldwork educator, and identify perceptions below.

Common perspectives between student and fieldwork educator	Different perspectives between student and fieldwork educator
Environment	
Fieldwork Educator	
Student	

2. What patterns are emerging across the three key components?

(Continued)

3. What strategies or changes can be implemented to promote a successful fieldwork experience? Describe below:

Components of a Successful Fieldwork	Environment, Fieldwork Educator and/or Student Strategies and Changes to Promote Successful Fieldwork Experience at This Setting
Environment Experiences Resources	
Fieldwork Educator Attidutes Behaviors Professional attributes	
Student Attitudes Behaviors	

This Fieldwork Experience Assessment Tool (FEAT) was developed by The Fieldwork Research Team: Karen Atler, Karmen Brown, Lou Ann Griswold, Wendy Krupnick, Luz Muniz de Melendez, and Patricia Stutz-Tanenbaum. Project funded by The American Occupational Therapy Foundation and AOTA Education Special Interest Section [April 1998; revised August 2001]

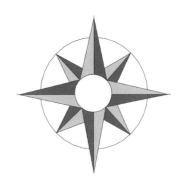

Appendix D.
Self-Assessment Tool for
Fieldwork Educator Competency

Fieldwork education is a vital component in preparing students for entering the practice of occupational therapy. This voluntary self-assessment tool establishes competency guidelines to facilitate the professional development of fieldwork educators from novice to experienced. This tool is designed to provide a structure for fieldwork educators to assess their own levels of competence to identify areas to pursue for developing and improving their skills. Competency as a fieldwork educator promotes the practitioner's pursuit of excellence in working with students to advance the profession.

Purpose

Both the novice and experienced COTA or OTR fieldwork educator can use the tool as an opportunity for self-reflection to target areas for professional growth. Proficiency as a fieldwork educator is an ongoing process of assessment, education, and practice. Fieldwork educators are continually working toward improving their proficiency in all competency areas as they supervise OTA/OT students. Use of this assessment tool is intended to be the foundation from which each fieldwork educator will create a professional growth plan with specific improvement strategies and measurable outcomes to advance professional development in this area of practice.

Content

- The self-assessment tool addresses fieldwork educator competencies in the areas of
  A. Professional practice
  B. Education
  C. Supervision
  D. Evaluation
  E. Administration.
- *Numerical Rating Scale:* Likert scale from 1 *(Low Proficiency)* to 5 *(High Proficiency)*.
- *Comment Section:* This section is intended to be used by the fieldwork educator to begin to identify aspects of competency for self-improvement.

- *Fieldwork Educator Professional Development Plan:* The plan is the outcome of the self-assessment. Fieldwork educators can use the suggested format for recording a professional development plan of action. The suggested format or chart may be copied for additional space.
- All fieldwork educators must meet the standards for fieldwork educator stated in the *Essentials and Guidelines for an Accredited Educational Program for the Occupational Therapist/Occupational Therapy Assistant.*
- *Terminology:* The terminology is based on a wide field of occupational therapy practice to address all fieldwork placement opportunities. For example, "individuals" is used to refer to consumers, patients, etc., served by occupational therapists and occupational therapy assistants.

Who Should Use the Tool?

This self-assessment tool is designed to be used by COTA and OTR fieldwork supervisors at all levels of expertise in educating students. While the tool is primarily oriented toward the COTA/OTR practitioner who directly supervises OTA and/or OT Level II Fieldwork, it can be applied to Level I Fieldwork and to non-OT supervisors.

Directions

- The fieldwork educator will determine the relevance of each competency to the role of the COTA/OTR in their setting. Some competency statements may not be applicable (COTA/OTR role delineation).
  - Self-Assessment Tool:
  - Circle the number that correlates with your level of competence for each item.
  - The Comment section can be used to highlight strengths, areas that need improvement, etc.
- Professional Development Plan:
  - It is helpful to prioritize the competency areas that need improvement
  - Select a few areas
  - Write goals for each of the selected areas
  - Identify strategies to meet the goals
  - Establish a deadline for meeting the goals
  - Comparing the actual date of completion to the target date may be helpful information to use when working on future development plans
- Allow time to complete the assessment tool and to create the professional development plan. It can be completed in one or more sessions.
- The tool is for personal use only. It should not be used as a performance appraisal. Fieldwork educators may, however, want to include goals from their professional development plan as a part of their annual professional goals.

OT practitioners are adept in assessing, planning, and implementing a practical and meaningful continuous quality improvement plan. It is this attribute plus a desire to support the growth of future practitioners that motivates COTAs and OTRs to seek methods for gaining and maintaining their competence as fieldwork educators. We hope this tool is helpful in guiding fieldwork educators on a journey of self-appraisal and professional development. Although it may only be a beginning step in developing standards of practice in fieldwork education, it meets the immediate need of defining basic competencies of fieldwork educators. It is in this spirit that the "Self-Assessment Tool" was drafted and offered as a means for better serving the needs of individuals and the future of Occupational Therapy.

The committee would like to acknowledge and thank the WISCOUNCIL (Wisconsin Council on Occupational Therapy Education) for their pioneer work in the development of this tool.

Nancy L. Beck, MA, OTR/L, *Task Force Chairperson*

Task Force Members: Claudia B. Brown, MS, OTR; Linda M. Kogut, MA, OTR; Patricia Stutz-Tanenbaum, MS, OTR; Marsha Zoll, OTR; Christine A. Bird, MA, OTR/L, *AOTA Liaison*

Self-Assessment Tool for Fieldwork Educator Competency

Key Definition Statement: *The fieldwork educator demonstrates competencies in professional knowledge, skills, and judgment in occupational therapy practice.*

A. Professional Practice Competencies

The fieldwork educator:	Low Proficient	Circle One		Highly Proficient	Comments
	1	←→		5	
1. Uses a systematic approach to evaluation and intervention based upon theory.	1	2	3	4	5	
2. Skillfully collects and analyzes evaluation and intervention data.	1	2	3	4	5	
3. Considers performance context, including temporal and environmental aspects, when determining feasibility and appropriateness of interventions.	1	2	3	4	5	
4. Objectively defines individual's problems.	1	2	3	4	5	
5. Articulates the rationale and theory base for occupational therapy intervention process (e.g., screening, evaluation, intervention planning, discharge planning).	1	2	3	4	5	
6. Collaborates with individuals, colleagues, family/support system, and other staff/professionals with respect, sensitivity, and professional judgment.	1	2	3	4	5	

A. Professional Practice Competencies	Key Definition Statement: *The fieldwork educator demonstrates competencies in professional knowledge, skills, and judgment in occupational therapy practice.*					
	Circle One					Comments
	Low Proficient				Highly Proficient	
	1 ←————→ 5					
The fieldwork educator:						
7. Works effectively with challenging interpersonal situations, (e.g., value differences, multi-cultural diversity, personality conflicts).	1	2	3	4	5	
8. Effectively manages and prioritizes practice (e.g., intervention, documentation, team meetings).	1	2	3	4	5	
9. Incorporates legal, ethical, and professional issues that influence practice (e.g., reimbursement, confidentiality, role delineation).	1	2	3	4	5	
10. Articulates and implements COTA/OTR role delineations as relevant to the practice setting.	1	2	3	4	5	
11. Adheres to professional practice standards.	1	2	3	4	5	
12. Assumes responsibility for and pursues professional development to expand knowledge and skills (e.g., understands own strengths and limitations).	1	2	3	4	5	

(Continued)

B. Education Competencies

Key Definition Statement: *The fieldwork educator facilitates the student's development of professional skills for entry-level practice. The fieldwork educator assumes responsibility for improving her/his skills as a fieldwork educator.*

	Circle One			Comments
	Low Proficient		Highly Proficient	
	1 ———————————————→ 5			
The fieldwork educator:				
1. Provides ongoing assessment of student's individual learning needs based on review of academic preparation, OTA and OT roles, prior experiences, and current performance level.	1 2	3	4 5	
2. Sequences learning experiences to grade progression toward entry-level practice.	1 2	3	4 5	
3. Facilitates student-directed learning within the parameters of the fieldwork environment.	1 2	3	4 5	
4. Maximizes opportunities for learning by using planned and unplanned experiences within the fieldwork environment.	1 2	3	4 5	
5. Uses a variety of instructional strategies to facilitate the learning process (e.g., role modeling, co-intervention, videotaping).	1 2	3	4 5	
6. Works effectively with all students, including those who have physical and/or psychosocial disability(s) and/or diverse age, gender, and multicultural characteristics.	1 2	3	4 5	

B. Education Competencies

Key Definition Statement: *The fieldwork educator facilitates the student's development of professional skills for entry-level practice. The fieldwork educator assumes responsibility for improving her/his skills as a fieldwork educator.*

B. Education Competencies	Circle One					Comments
	Low Proficient			Highly Proficient		
The fieldwork educator:	1 ———————————————————→ 5					
7. Guides student integration of therapeutic concepts and skills (e.g., promotes student discussion to elicit clinical reasoning for selected intervention and/or to process personal feelings/values that interface with practice).	1	2	3	4	5	
8. Self-identifies and implements a Fieldwork Educator Professional Development Plan. (See page 8 for suggested plan.)	1	2	3	4	5	
9. Identifies resources to promote student and fieldwork educator professional development (e.g., academic program, student and supervisor mentors, AOTA Education Department, Commission on Education, Education Special Interest Section, workshops, inservices).	1	2	3	4	5	
10. Provides reference materials to promote student and fieldwork educator professional development (e.g., publications, texts, videos, Internet).	1	2	3	4	5	

(Continued)

C. Supervision Competencies

Key Definition Statement: *The fieldwork educator monitors and guides student achievement of entry-level practice.*

Supervision Competencies	Circle One — Low Proficient 1 ←→ 5 Highly Proficient					Comments
The fieldwork educator:						
1. Presents clear performance expectations initially and throughout the experience appropriate to OT practice (e.g., student OTA/OT role delineation, Level I/II Fieldwork, practice environment).	1	2	3	4	5	
2. Collaborates with the student in setting learning goals, objectives, and expectations and makes modifications accordingly.	1	2	3	4	5	
3. Anticipates and prepares student for challenging situations.	1	2	3	4	5	
4. Provides activities to challenge student's optimal performance.	1	2	3	4	5	
5. Provides the student with prompt, direct, specific, and constructive feedback throughout the fieldwork experience.	1	2	3	4	5	
6. Makes specific suggestions to the student for improvement in performance.	1	2	3	4	5	

Key Definition Statement: *The fieldwork educator monitors and guides student achievement of entry-level practice.*

C. Supervision Competencies	Circle One					Comments
	Low Proficient				Highly Proficient	
	1				5	
The fieldwork educator:						
7. Uses verbal, nonverbal, and written communication effectively.	1	2	3	4	5	
8. Initiates interaction to resolve conflict and to raise issues of concern.	1	2	3	4	5	
9. Uses a variety of supervisory approaches to facilitate student performance (e.g., written, support/confrontation, multiple supervisors).	1	2	3	4	5	
10. Elicits and responds to student's feedback and concerns.	1	2	3	4	5	
11. Collaborates with the student and academic fieldwork coordinator to identify and modify learning situations when student experiences difficulty.	1	2	3	4	5	
12. Acts as a role model of professional behavior (e.g., separates personal versus professional issues with students and staff, addresses diversity issues, uses a sense of humor appropriately).	1	2	3	4	5	

(Continued)

D. Evaluation Competencies

Key Definition Statement: *The fieldwork educator evaluates student performance for achievement of entry-level practice.*

The fieldwork educator:

	Low Proficient	Circle One	Highly Proficient		Comments
	1 ←——→ 5				
1. Reviews with student the evaluation tool and expected entry-level standards (e.g., behavioral objectives, weekly objectives) to be used at midterm and final evaluation.	1	2	3	4	5
2. Assesses student according to performance standards based on objective information (e.g., direct observation, discussion with student, review of student's documentation, observation by others).	1	2	3	4	5
3. Assesses student's performance based on appropriate COTA/OTR entry-level roles of the fieldwork setting.	1	2	3	4	5
4. Involves the student in self-reflection and self-assessment during the evaluation process.	1	2	3	4	5
5. Uses evaluation process to counsel student on strengths and opportunities for growth.	1	2	3	4	5

226

D. Evaluation Competencies	Key Definition Statement: *The fieldwork educator evaluates student performance for achievement of entry-level practice.*					
	Circle One					Comments
	Low Proficient				Highly Proficient	
	1 $\longrightarrow$				5	
The fieldwork educator:						
6. Uses fieldwork evaluation tools to accurately measure student performance.	1	2	3	4	5	
7. Completes and distributes in a timely manner all evaluations regarding student performance, including but not limited to the midterm and final evaluation (e.g., AOTA Fieldwork Evaluation).	1	2	3	4	5	
8. Guides the student in the use of the performance evaluation as a method of promoting continued professional growth and development.	1	2	3	4	5	
9. Documents student's fieldwork performance recognizing ethical and legal rights (e.g., due process, confidentiality, ADA, integrity).	1	2	3	4	5	

(Continued)

227

E. Administration Competencies

Key Definition Statement: The fieldwork educator develops and/or implements an organized program in keeping with legal/professional standards and environmental factors (physical, social, and cultural).

	Circle One					Comments
	Low Proficient				Highly Proficient	
The fieldwork educator:	1 ←———————→ 5					
1. Communicates and collaborates with academic programs (e.g., fieldwork agreement, confirmation, student placement).	1	2	3	4	5	
2. Seeks support from fieldwork site administration and staff for the student program.	1	2	3	4	5	
3. Designs and/or implements the fieldwork program in compliance with professional standards (e.g., AOTA *Essentials*, academic and fieldwork setting requirements, Standards of Practice, Code of Ethics).	1	2	3	4	5	
4. Assures that the fieldwork program is sensitive to diversity and multi-cultural issues.	1	2	3	4	5	
5. Documents an organized, systematic fieldwork program (e.g., fieldwork manual, student expectations, weekly sequence).	1	2	3	4	5	
6. Documents behavioral objectives to achieve fieldwork goals appropriate for COTA/OTR entry-level practice.	1	2	3	4	5	

E. Administration Competencies	Key Definition Statement: *The fieldwork educator develops and/or implements an organized program in keeping with legal/professional standards and environmental factors (physical, social, and cultural).*					
	Circle One					Comments
	Low Proficient				Highly Proficient	
The fieldwork educator:	1 ⟶ 5					
7. Defines essential functions and roles of a fieldwork student, in compliance with legal and accreditation standards (e.g., ADA, Family Education Rights and Privacy Act, fieldwork agreement, reimbursement mechanism, state regulations).	1	2	3	4	5	
8. Provides student work areas appropriate to fieldwork site (e.g., student safety, accessibility, supplies).	1	2	3	4	5	
9. Provides a complete orientation for student to fieldwork site (e.g., policies, procedures, student expectations, and responsibilities).	1	2	3	4	5	
10. Requires student compliance with the fieldwork site mission, goals, philosophy, and standards.	1	2	3	4	5	
11. Submits required fieldwork documents to academic program in a timely manner (e.g., fieldwork evaluation, fieldwork agreements, fieldwork data form).	1	2	3	4	5	
12. Conducts ongoing fieldwork program evaluations and monitors changes in the program with student and staff input (e.g., Student Evaluation of Fieldwork Experience, Self-Assessment Tool for Fieldwork Competencies).	1	2	3	4	5	

(Continued)

Fieldwork Educator Professional Development Plan

Name: _____

Date: _____

Strengths: _____
_____
_____
_____

Areas to Develop: _____
_____
_____
_____

Strategies to Improve Competency

Competency Area to Address	Goals	Independent Study	Academic Coursework	Workshops/Continuing Education	Student Feedback	Consult With Academic Fieldwork Coordinator	Presentations	Publications	Research Activities	Mentorship	Peer Review	Shared Supervision of Student			Target Date	Completed Date

Note. You are welcome to make additional copies of this chart.

Adapted from: *Developing, maintaining, and updating competency in occupational therapy: A guide to self-appraisal. AOTA, 1995*

American Occupational Therapy Association, Inc., COE Fieldwork Issues Committee, 11/97

American Occupational Therapy Association Reference List

American Occupational Therapy Association. *Developing, maintaining, and updating competency in occupational therapy: A guide to self-appraisal.* Bethesda, MD: Author, 1995.

American Occupational Therapy Association. *Educating college students with disabilities: What academic and fieldwork educators need to know.* Bethesda, MD: Author, 1997.

American Occupational Therapy Association. *Essentials and guidelines for an accredited educational program for the occupational therapist.* Bethesda, MD: Author, 1991.

American Occupational Therapy Association. *Essentials and guidelines for an accredited educational program for the occupational therapy assistant.* Bethesda, MD: Author, 1991.

American Occupational Therapy Association. *Guide to fieldwork education.* Bethesda, MD: Author, 1993.

American Occupational Therapy Association. *Occupational therapy code of ethics.* Bethesda, MD: Author, 1994.

American Occupational Therapy Association. *Occupational therapy roles and career exploration and development: A companion guide to the occupational therapy roles document.* Bethesda, MD: Author, 1994.

American Occupational Therapy Association. *Standards of practice for occupational therapy.* Bethesda, MD: Author, 1994.

American Occupational Therapy Association. *Uniform terminology for occupational therapy-third edition.* Bethesda, MD: Author, 1994.

Crepeau, E. B. and LaGarde, T, (eds). *Self-paced instruction for clinical education and supervision.* Bethesda, MD: AOTA, 1991.

Frum, D. and Opacich, K. Supervision: *Development of therapeutic competence.* Bethesda, MD: AOTA, 1987.

Meyers, S. and Swinehart, S. *Creating a positive level I fieldwork experience.* Bethesda, MD: AOTA, 1995.

Smith, V. *Occupational therapy: Transition from classroom to clinic-Physical disability fieldwork applications.* Bethesda, MD: AOTA, 1994.

Acknowledgment: Thanks to WISCOUNCIL (Wisconsin Council on Occupational Therapy Education) for their pioneer work in the development of this tool.

Additional resources available through AOTA:
• Regional Fieldwork Consultants Network
• Education Special Interest Section
• AOTA's Education Department.

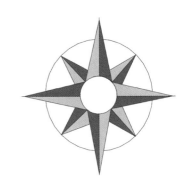

Appendix E.
Occupational Therapy
Code of Ethics (2005)

Preamble

The American Occupational Therapy Association (AOTA) *Occupational Therapy Code of Ethics (2005)* is a public statement of principles used to promote and maintain high standards of conduct within the profession and is supported by the *Core Values and Attitudes of Occupational Therapy Practice* (AOTA, 1993). Members of AOTA are committed to promoting inclusion, diversity, independence, and safety for all recipients in various stages of life, health, and illness and to empower all beneficiaries of occupational therapy. This commitment extends beyond service recipients to include professional colleagues, students, educators, businesses, and the community.

Fundamental to the mission of the occupational therapy profession is the therapeutic use of everyday life activities (occupations) with individuals or groups for the purpose of participation in roles and situations in home, school, workplace, community, and other settings. "Occupational therapy addresses the physical, cognitive, psychosocial, sensory, and other aspects of performance in a variety of contexts to support engagement in everyday life activities that affect health, well-being and quality of life" (*Definition of Occupational Therapy Practice for the AOTA Model Practice Act,* 2004). Occupational therapy personnel have an ethical responsibility first and foremost to recipients of service as well as to society.

The historical foundation of this Code is based on ethical reasoning surrounding practice and professional issues, as well as empathic reflection regarding these interactions with others. This reflection resulted in the establishment of principles that guide ethical action. Ethical action goes beyond rote following of rules or application of principles; rather, it is a manifestation of moral character and mindful reflection. It is a commitment to beneficence for the sake of others, to virtuous practice of artistry and science, to genuinely good behaviors, and to noble acts of courage. It is an empathic way of being among others, which is made every day by all occupational therapy personnel.

The AOTA *Occupational Therapy Code of Ethics (2005)* is an aspirational guide to professional conduct when ethical issues surface. Ethical decision making is a process that includes awareness regarding how the outcome will impact occupational therapy clients in all spheres. Applications of Code principles are considered situation-specific, and where a conflict exists, occupational therapy personnel will pursue responsible efforts for resolution.

The specific purpose of the AOTA *Occupational Therapy Code of Ethics (2005)* is to:

1. Identify and describe the principles supported by the occupational therapy profession
2. Educate the general public and members regarding established principles to which occupational therapy personnel are accountable
3. Socialize occupational therapy personnel new to the practice to expected standards of conduct
4. Assist occupational therapy personnel in recognition and resolution of ethical dilemmas.

The AOTA *Occupational Therapy Code of Ethics* (2005) defines the set principles that apply to occupational therapy personnel at all levels:

Principle 1. Occupational therapy personnel shall demonstrate a concern for the safety and well-being of the recipients of their services. (BENEFICENCE)

Occupational therapy personnel shall

A. Provide services in a fair and equitable manner. They shall recognize and appreciate the cultural components of economics, geography, race, ethnicity, religious and political factors, marital status, age, sexual orientation, gender identity, and disability of all recipients of their services.
B. Strive to ensure that fees are fair and reasonable and commensurate with services performed. When occupational therapy practitioners set fees, they shall set fees considering institutional, local, state, and federal requirements, and with due regard for the service recipient's ability to pay.
C. Make every effort to advocate for recipients to obtain needed services through available means.
D. Recognize the responsibility to promote public health and the safety and well-being of individuals, groups, and/or communities.

Principle 2. Occupational therapy personnel shall take measures to ensure a recipient's safety and avoid imposing or inflicting harm. (NONMALEFICENCE)

Occupational therapy personnel shall

A. Maintain therapeutic relationships that shall not exploit the recipient of services sexually, physically, emotionally, psychologically, financially, socially, or in any other manner.

B. Avoid relationships or activities that conflict or interfere with therapeutic professional judgment and objectivity.

C. Refrain from any undue influences that may compromise provision of service.

D. Exercise professional judgment and critically analyze directives that could result in potential harm before implementation.

E. Identify and address personal problems that may adversely impact professional judgment and duties.

F. Bring concerns regarding impairment of professional skills of a colleague to the attention of the appropriate authority when or if attempts to address concerns are unsuccessful.

Principle 3. Occupational therapy personnel shall respect recipients to assure their rights. (AUTONOMY, CONFIDENTIALITY)

Occupational therapy personnel shall

A. Collaborate with recipients, and if theydesire, families, significant others, and/or caregivers in setting goals and priorities throughout the intervention process, including full disclosure of the nature, risk, and potential outcomes of any interventions.

B. Obtain informed consent from participants involved in research activities and ensure that they understand potential risks and outcomes.

C. Respect the individual's right to refuse professional services or involvement in research or educational activities.

D. Protect all privileged confidential forms of written, verbal, and electronic communication gained from educational, practice, research, and investigational activities unless otherwise mandated by local, state, or federal regulations.

Principle 4. Occupational therapy personnel shall achieve and continually maintain high standards of competence. (DUTY)

Occupational therapy personnel shall

A. Hold the appropriate national, state, or any other requisite credentials for the services they provide.

B. Conform to AOTA standards of practice and official documents.

C. Take responsibility for maintaining and documenting competence in practice, education, and research by participating in professional development and educational activities.

D. Be competent in all topic areas in which they provide instruction to consumers, peers, and/or students.

E. Critically examine available evidence so they may perform their duties on the basis of current information.

F. Protect service recipients by ensuring that duties assumed by or assigned to other occupational therapy personnel match credentials, qualifications, experience, and scope of practice.

G. Provide appropriate supervision to individuals for whom they have supervisory responsibility in accordance with Association official documents; local, state, and federal or national laws and regulations; and institutional policies and procedures.

H. Refer to or consult with other service providers whenever such a referral or consultation would be helpful to the care of the recipient of service. The referral or consultation process shall be done in collaboration with the recipient of service.

Principle 5. Occupational therapy personnel shall comply with laws and Association policies guiding the profession of occupational therapy. (PROCEDURAL JUSTICE)

Occupational therapy personnel shall

A. Familiarize themselves with and seek to understand and abide by institutional rules; applicable Association policies; and local, state, and federal/national/international laws.

B. Be familiar with revisions in those laws and Association policies that apply to the profession of occupational therapy and shall inform employers, employees, and colleagues of those changes.

C. Encourage those they supervise in occupational therapy–related activities to adhere to the Code.

D. Take reasonable steps to ensure employers are aware of occupational therapy's ethical obligations, as set forth in this Code, and of the implications of those obligations for occupational therapy practice, education, and research.

E. Record and report in an accurate and timely manner all information related to professional activities.

Principle 6. Occupational therapy personnel shall provide accurate information when representing the profession. (VERACITY)

Occupational therapy personnel shall

A. Represent their credentials, qualifications, education, experience, training, and competence accurately. This is of particular importance for those to whom occupational therapy personnel provide their services or with whom occupational therapy personnel have a professional relationship.

B. Disclose any professional, personal, financial, business, or volunteer affiliations that may pose a conflict of interest to those with whom they may establish a professional, contractual, or other working relationship.

C. Refrain from using or participating in the use of any form of communication that contains false, fraudulent, deceptive, or unfair statements or claims.

D. Identify and fully disclose to all appropriate persons errors that compromise recipients' safety.

E. Accept responsibility for their professional actions that reduce the public's trust in occupational therapy services and those that perform those services.

Principle 7. Occupational therapy personnel shall treat colleagues and other professionals with respect, fairness, discretion, and integrity. (FIDELITY)

Occupational therapy personnel shall

A. Preserve, respect, and safeguard confidential information about colleagues and staff, unless otherwise mandated by national, state, or local laws.

B. Accurately represent the qualifications, views, contributions, and findings of colleagues.

C. Take adequate measures to discourage, prevent, expose, and correct any breaches of the Code and report any breaches of the Code to the appropriate authority.

D. Avoid conflicts of interest and conflicts of commitment in employment and volunteer roles.

E. Use conflict resolution and/or alternative dispute resolution resources to resolve organizational and interpersonal conflicts.

F. Familiarize themselves with established policies and procedures for handling concerns about this Code, including familiarity with national, state, local, district, and territorial procedures for handling ethics complaints. These include policies and procedures created by AOTA, licensing and regulatory bodies, employers, agencies, certification boards, and other organizations having jurisdiction over occupational therapy practice.

Glossary

Autonomy
The right of an individual to self-determination. The ability to independently act on one's decisions for one's own well-being (Beauchamp & Childress, 2001).

Beneficence
Doing good for others or bringing about good for them. The duty to confer benefits to others.

Confidentiality
Not disclosing data or information that should be kept private to prevent harm and to abide by policies, regulations, and laws.

Dilemma
A situation in which one moral conviction or right action conflicts with another. It exists because there is no one, clear-cut, right answer.

Duty
Actions required of professionals by society or actions that are self-imposed.

Ethics
A systematic study of morality (i.e., rules of conduct that are grounded in philosophical principles and theory).

Fidelity
Faithfully fulfilling vows and promises, agreements, and discharging fiduciary responsibilities (Beauchamp & Childress, 2001).

Justice
Three types of justice are
- **Compensatory justice**—Making reparation for wrongs that have been done.
- **Distributive justice**—The act of distributing goods and burdens among members of society.
- **Procedural justice**—Assuring that processes are organized in a fair manner and policies or laws are followed.

Morality
Personal beliefs regarding values, rules, and principles of what is right or wrong. Morality may be culture-based or culture-driven.

Nonmaleficence

Not harming or causing harm to be done to oneself or others; the duty to ensure that no harm is done.

Veracity

A duty to tell the truth; avoid deception.

References

American Occupational Therapy Association. (1993). Core values and attitudes of occupational therapy practice. *American Journal of Occupational Therapy, 47,* 1085–1086.

American Occupational Therapy Association. (1998). Guidelines to the occupational therapy code of ethics. *American Journal of Occupational Therapy, 52,* 881–884.

American Occupational Therapy Association. (2004). Association policies. *American Journal of Occupational Therapy, 58,* 694–695.

Beauchamp, T. L., & Childress, J. F. (2001). *Principles of biomedical ethics* (5th ed.). New York: Oxford University Press.

Definition of Occupational Therapy Practice forthe AOTA Model Practice Act. (2004). Retrieved April 9, 2005, from www.aota.org/members/area4/docs/defotpractice.pdf

Authors

Commission on Standards and Ethics (SEC):

S. Maggie Reitz, PhD, OTR/L, FAOTA, *Chairperson*
Melba Arnold, MS, OTR/L
Linda Gabriel Franck, PhD, OTR/L
Darryl J. Austin, MS, OT/L
Diane Hill, COTA/L, AP, ROH
Lorie J. McQuade, MEd, CRC
Daryl K. Knox, MD
Deborah Yarett Slater, MS, OT/L, FAOTA, *Staff Liaison*

With contributions to the Preamble by

Suzanne Peloquin, PhD, OTR, FAOTA

Adopted by the RepresentativeAssembly 2005C202

Note. This document replaces the 2000 document, *Occupational Therapy Code of Ethics (2000) (American Journal of Occupational Therapy, 54,* 614–616).

Prepared 4/7/2000, revised draft 1/2005, second revision 4/2005 by SEC.

Note: Commission on Standards and Ethics (SEC) changed to Ethics Commission (EC) in September 2005 per AOTA Bylaws.

Note. This *AOTA Occupational Therapy Code of Ethics* is one of three documents that constitute the "Ethics Standards." The other two are the *Core Values and Attitudes of Occupational Therapy Practice* (1993) and the *Guidelines to the Occupational Therapy Code of Ethics.*

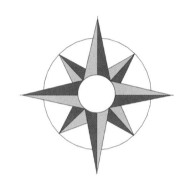

Appendix F.
Guidelines to the Occupational Therapy Code of Ethics

Professional Behaviors	Principles From Code
1. Honesty: *Professionals must be honest with themselves, must be honest with all whom they come in contact with, and must know their strengths and limitations.*	
1.1. In education, research, practice, and leadership roles, individuals must \be honest in receiving and disseminating information by providing opportunities for informed consent and for discussion of available options.	Veracity
1.2. Occupational therapy practitioners must be certain that informed consent has been obtained prior to the initiation of services, including evaluation. If the service recipient cannot give informed consent, the practitioner must be sure that consent has been obtained from the person who is legally responsible for the service recipient.	Autonomy, Veracity
1.3. Occupational therapy practitioners must be truthful about their individual competencies as well as the competence of those under their supervision. In some cases the therapist may need to refer the client to another professional to assure that the most appropriate services are provided.	Duty, Veracity
1.4. Referrals to other health care specialists shall be based exclusively on the other provider's competence and ability to provide the needed service.	Beneficence
1.5. All documentation must accurately reflect the nature and quantity of services provided.	Veracity
1.6. Occupational therapy practitioners terminate services when they do not meet the needs and goals of the recipient or when services no longer produce a measurable outcome.	Procedural Justice, Beneficence
1.7. All marketing and advertising must be truthful and carefully presented to avoid misleading the client or the public.	Veracity

(Continued)

Professional Behaviors	Principles From Code
1.8. All occupational therapy personnel shall accurately represent their credentials and roles.	Veracity
1.9. Occupational therapy personnel shall not use funds for unintended purposes or misappropriate funds.	Duty, Veracity
2. Communication: *Communication is important in all aspects of occupational therapy. Individuals must be conscientious and truthful in all facets of written, verbal, and electronic communication.*	
2.1. Occupational therapy personnel do not make deceptive, fraudulent, or misleading statements about the nature of the services they provide or the outcomes that can be expected.	Veracity
2.2. Professional contracts for occupational therapy services shall explicitly describe the type and duration of services as well as the duties and responsibilities of all involved parties.	Veracity, Procedural Justice
2.3. Documentation for reimbursement purposes shall be done in accordance with applicable laws, guidelines, and regulations.	Veracity, Procedural Justice
2.4. Documentation shall accurately reflect the services delivered and the outcomes. It shall be of the kind and quality that satisfies the scrutiny of peer reviews, legal proceedings, payers, regulatory bodies, and accrediting agencies.	Veracity, Procedural Justice, Duties
2.5. Occupational therapy personnel must be honest in gathering and giving fact-based information regarding job performance and fieldwork performance. Information given shall be timely and truthful, accurate, and respectful of all parties involved.	Veracity, Fidelity
2.6. Documentation for supervisory purposes shall accurately reflect the factual components of the interactions and the expected outcomes.	Veracity
2.7. Occupational therapy personnel must give credit and recognition when using the work of others.	Veracity, Procedural Justice
2.8. Occupational therapy personnel do not fabricate data, falsify information, or plagiarize.	Veracity, Procedural Justice
2.9. Occupational therapy personnel refrain from using biased or derogatory language in written, verbal, and electronic communication about clients, students, research participants, and colleagues.	Nonmaleficence, Fidelity

Professional Behaviors	Principles From Code
2.10. Occupational therapy personnel who provide information through oral and written means shall emphasize that ethical and appropriate service delivery for clients cannot be done without proper individualized evaluations and plans of care.	Beneficence
3. Ensuring the Common Good: *Occupational therapy personnel are expected to increase awareness of the profession's social responsibilities to help ensure the common good.*	
3.1. Occupational therapy personnel take steps to make sure that employers are aware of the ethical principles of the profession and occupational therapy personnel's obligation to adhere to those ethical principles.	Duty
3.2. Occupational therapy personnel shall be diligent stewards of human, financial, and material resources of their employers. They shall refrain from exploiting these resources for personal gain.	Fidelity
3.3. Occupational therapy personnel should actively work with their employer to prevent discrimination and unfair labor practices. They should also advocate for employees with disabilities to ensure the provision of reasonable accommodations.	Procedural Justice
3.4. Occupational therapy personnel should actively participate with their employer in the formulation of policies and procedures. They should do this to ensure that these policies and procedures are legal, in accordance with regulations governing aspects of practice, and consistent with the AOTA Occupational Therapy Code of Ethics.	Procedural Justice
3.5. Occupational therapy personnel in educational settings are responsible for promoting ethical conduct by students, faculty, and fieldwork colleagues.	Duty, Fidelity
3.6. Occupational therapy personnel involved in or preparing to be involved in research, including education and policy research, need to obtain all necessary approvals prior to initiating research.	Procedural Justice
4. Competence: *Occupational therapy personnel are expected to work within their areas of competence and to pursue opportunities to update, increase, and expand their competence.*	
4.1. Occupational therapy personnel developing new areas of competence (skills, techniques, approaches) must engage in appropriate study and training, under appropriate supervision, before incorporating new areas into their practice.	Duty

(Continued)

243

Professional Behaviors	Principles From Code
4.2. When generally recognized standards do not exist in emerging areas of practice, occupational therapy personnel must take responsible steps to ensure their own competence.	Duty
4.3. Occupational therapy personnel shall develop an understanding and appreciation for different cultures in order to be able to provide culturally competent service. Culturally competent practitioners are aware of how service delivery can be affected by economic, age, ethnic, racial, geographic, gender, gender identity, religious, and political factors, as well as marital status, sexual orientation, and disability.	Beneficence, Duty
4.4. In areas where the ability to communicate with the client is limited (e.g., aphasia, different language, literacy), occupational therapy personnel shall take appropriate steps to facilitate meaningful communication and comprehension.	Autonomy
4.5. Occupational therapy personnel must ensure that skilled occupational therapy interventions or techniques are performed only by qualified persons.	Duty, Beneficence, Nonmaleficence
4.6. Occupational therapy administrators (academic, research, and clinical) are responsible for ensuring the competence and qualifications of personnel in their employment.	Beneficence, Nonmaleficence
5. Confidential and Protected Information: *Information that is confidential must remain confidential. This information cannot be shared verbally, electronically, or in writing without appropriate consent. Information must be shared on a need-to-know basis only with those having primary responsibilities for decision making.*	
5.1. All occupational therapy personnel shall respect the confidential nature of information gained in any occupational therapy interaction. The only exceptions are when a practitioner or staff member believes that an individual is in serious, foreseeable, or imminent harm. In this instance, laws and regulations require disclosure to appropriate authorities without consent.	Confidentiality
5.2. Occupational therapy personnel shall respect the clients' and colleagues' right to privacy.	Confidentiality
5.3. Occupational therapy personnel shall maintain the confidentiality of all verbal, written, electronic, augmentative, and non-verbal communications (as required by HIPAA).	Confidentiality

Professional Behaviors	Principles From Code
6. Conflict of Interest: *Avoidance of real or perceived conflict of interest is imperative to maintaining the integrity of interactions.*	
6.1. Occupational therapy personnel shall be alert to and avoid any action that would interfere with the exercise of impartial professional judgment during the delivery of occupational therapy services.	Nonmaleficence
6.2. Occupational therapy personnel shall not take advantage of or exploit anyone to further their own personal interests.	Nonmaleficence
6.3. Gifts and remuneration from individuals, agencies, or companies must be reported in accordance with employer policies as well as state and federal guidelines.	Veracity, Procedural Justice
6.4. Occupational therapy personnel shall not accept obligations or duties that may compete with or be in conflict with their duties to their employers.	Veracity, Fidelity
6.5. Occupational therapy personnel shall not use their position or the knowledge gained from their position in such a way that knowingly gives rise to real or perceived conflict of interest between themselves and their employers, other association members or bodies, and/or other organizations.	Veracity, Fidelity
7. Impaired Practitioner: *Occupational therapy personnel who cannot competently perform their duties after reasonable accommodation are considered to be impaired. The occupational therapy practitioner's basic duty to students, patients, colleagues, and research subjects is to ensure that no harm is done. It is difficult to report a professional colleague who is impaired. The motive for this action must be to provide for the protection and safety of all, including the person who is impaired.*	
7.1. Occupational therapy personnel shall be aware of their own personal problems and limitations that may interfere with their ability to perform their job competently. They should know when these problems have the potential to cause harm to clients, colleagues, students, research participants, or others.	Nonmaleficence
7.2. The individual should seek the appropriate professional help and take steps to remedy personal problems and limitations that interfere with job performance.	Nonmaleficence
7.3. Occupational therapy personnel who believe that a colleague's impairment interferes with safe and effective practice should, when possible, discuss their questions and concerns with the individual and assist their colleague in seeking appropriate help or treatment.	Nonmaleficence

(Continued)

Professional Behaviors	Principles From Code
7.4. When efforts to assist an impaired colleague fail, the occupational therapy practitioner is responsible for reporting the individual to the appropriate authority (e.g., employer, agency, licensing or regulatory board, certification body, professional organization).	Nonmaleficence
8. Sexual Relationships: *Sexual relationships that occur during any professional interaction are forms of misconduct.*	
8.1. Because of potential coercion or harm to former clients, students, or research participants, occupational therapy practitioners are responsible for ensuring that the individual with whom they enter into a romantic/sexual relationship has not been coerced or exploited in any way.	Nonmaleficence
8.2. Sexual relationships with current clients, employees, students, or research participants are not permissible, even if the relationship is consensual.	Nonmaleficence
8.3. Occupational therapy personnel must not sexually harass any persons.	Nonmaleficence
8.4. Occupational therapy personnel have full responsibility to set clear and appropriate boundaries in their professional interactions.	Nonmaleficence
9. Payment for Services and Other Financial Arrangements: *Occupational therapy personnel shall not guarantee or promise specific outcomes for occupational therapy services. Payment for occupational therapy services shall not be contingent on successful outcomes.*	
9.1. Occupational therapy personnel shall only collect fees legally. Fees shall be fair and reasonable and commensurate with services delivered.	Procedural Justice
9.2. Occupational therapy personnel do not ordinarily participate in bartering for services because of potential exploitation and conflict of interest. However, such an arrangement may be appropriate if it is not clinically contraindicated, if the relationship is not exploitative, and if bartering is a culturally appropriate custom.	Beneficence

Professional Behaviors	Principles From Code
9.3. Occupational therapy practitioners can render pro bono ("for the good," free of charge) or reduced-fee occupational therapy services for selected individuals only when consistent with guidelines of the business/facility, third-party payer, or government agency.	Beneficence, Procedural Justice
9.4. Occupational therapy personnel may engage in volunteer activities to improve access to occupational therapy or by providing individual service and expertise to charitable organizations.	Beneficence
9.5. Occupational therapy personnel who participate in a business arrangement as owner, stockholder, partner, or employee have an obligation to maintain the ethical principles and standards of the profession. They also shall refrain from working for or doing business with organizations that engage in illegal or unethical business practices (e.g., fraudulent billing).	Procedural Justice
10. **Resolving Ethical Issues:** *Occupational therapy personnel should utilize any and all resources available to them to identify and resolve conflicts and/or ethical dilemmas.*	
10.1. Occupational therapy personnel are obligated to be familiar with the Code and its application to their respective work environments. Occupational therapy practitioners are expected to share the Code with their employer and other employees and colleagues. Lack of familiarity with and knowledge of the Code is not an excuse or a defense against a charge of ethical misconduct.	Duty
10.2. Occupational therapy personnel who are uncertain of whether a specific action would violate the Code have a responsibility to consult with knowledgeable individuals, ethics committees, or other appropriate authorities.	Duty
10.3. When conflicts occur in professional organizations, members must clarify the nature of the conflict and, where possible, seek to resolve the conflict in a way that permits the fullest adherence to the Code.	Fidelity
10.4. Occupational therapy personnel shall attempt to resolve perceived violations of the Code within institutions by utilizing internal resources.	Fidelity

(Continued)

Professional Behaviors	Principles From Code
10.5. If the informal resolution is not appropriate or is not effective, the next step is to take action by consultation with or referral to institutional, local, district, territorial, state, or national groups who have jurisdiction over occupational therapy practice.	Fidelity
10.6. Occupational therapy personnel shall cooperate with ethics committee proceedings and comply with resulting requirements. Failure to cooperate is, in itself, an ethical violation.	Procedural Justice
10.7. Occupational therapy personnel shall file only formal ethics complaints aimed at protecting the public or promoting professional conduct rather than harming or discrediting a colleague.	Fidelity

Appendix G.
Standards for Continuing Competence

AOTA's Standards for Continuing Competence

Continuing competence is a process involving the examination of current competence and the development of capacity for the future. It is a component of ongoing professional development and lifelong learning. Continuing competence is a dynamic, multidimensional process in which the occupational therapist and occupational therapy assistant develop and maintain the knowledge, performance skills, interpersonal abilities, critical reasoning, and ethical reasoning skills necessary to perform current and future roles and responsibilities within the profession.

Occupational therapists and occupational therapy assistants use these standards to assess, maintain, and document continuing competence. Basic to these standards is the belief that all occupational therapists and occupational therapy assistants share core values and knowledge guiding actions within their roles and responsibilities. The core of occupational therapy involves an understanding of occupation and purposeful activities and their influence on human performance. Occupational therapists and occupational therapy assistants have unique skills in activity analysis and activity synthesis and in critical and ethical reasoning. The profession is based on the values of client-centered holistic intervention and the right of an individual to be self-determining.

Standard 1. Knowledge

Occupational therapists and occupational therapy assistants shall demonstrate understanding and comprehension of the information required for the multiple roles and responsibilities they assume. The individual must demonstrate

- Mastery of the core of occupational therapy as it is applied in the multiple responsibilities assumed;
- Expertise associated with primary responsibilities;
- Integration of relevant evidence, literature, and epidemiological data related to primary responsibilities and to the consumer population(s) served; and
- Integration of current Association documents and legislative, legal, and regulatory issues into practice.

Standard 2. Critical Reasoning

Occupational therapists and occupational therapy assistants shall use reasoning processes to make sound judgments and decisions. The individual must demonstrate

- Deductive and inductive reasoning in making decisions specific to roles and responsibilities;
- Problem-solving skills necessary to carry out responsibilities;
- The ability to analyze occupational performance as influenced by environmental factors;
- The ability to reflect on one's own practice;
- Management and synthesis of information from a variety of sources in support of making decisions; and
- Application of evidence, research findings, and outcome data in making decisions.

Standard 3. Interpersonal Abilities

Occupational therapists and occupational therapy assistants shall develop and maintain their professional relationships with others within the context of their roles and responsibilities. The individual must demonstrate

- Use of effective communication methods that match the abilities, personal factors, learning styles, and therapeutic needs of consumers and others;
- Effective interaction with people from diverse backgrounds;
- Use of feedback from consumers, families, supervisors, and colleagues to modify one's professional behavior;
- Collaboration with consumers, families, and professionals to attain optimal consumer outcomes; and
- The ability to develop and sustain team relationships to meet identified outcomes.

Standard 4. Performance Skills

Occupational therapists and occupational therapy assistants shall demonstrate the expertise, aptitudes, proficiencies, and abilities to competently fulfill their roles and responsibilities. The individual must demonstrate expertise in

- Practice grounded in the core of occupational therapy;
- The therapeutic use of self, the therapeutic use of occupations and activities, the consultation process, and the education process to bring about change;
- Integrating current practice techniques and technologies;
- Updating performance based on current research and literature; and

- Quality improvement processes that prevent practice error and maximize client outcomes.

Standard 5. Ethical Reasoning

Occupational therapists and occupational therapy assistants shall identify, analyze, and clarify ethical issues or dilemmas to make responsible decisions within the changing context of their roles and responsibilities. The individual must demonstrate

- Understanding and adherence to the profession's *Code of Ethics,* other relevant codes of ethics, and applicable laws and regulations;
- The use of ethical principles and the profession's core values to understand complex situations; and
- The integrity to make and defend decisions based on ethical reasoning.

Authors

The Commission on Continuing Competence and Professional Development
Penelope Moyers, EdD, OTR/L, BCMH, FAOTA, *Chairperson*
Jane Case-Smith, EdD, OT/L, BCP, FAOTA
Mary Kay Currie, OT, BCPR
Coralie H. Glantz, OT/L, BCG, FAOTA
Jim Hinojosa, OT, PhD, BCP, FAOTA
Maria Elena E. Louch, OT/L, *AOTA Headquarters Liaison*

for

The Commission on Continuing Competence and Professional Development
Penelope Moyers, EdD, OTR/L, FAOTA, *Chairperson*

Adopted by the Representative Assembly 2005C243

Edited 2006

This document replaces the 1999 document *Standards for Continuing Competence (American Journal of Occupational Therapy, 53,* 559–560).

Copyright © 2005, by the American Occupational Therapy Association. Previously published in the *American Journal of Occupational Therapy, 59,* 661–662.

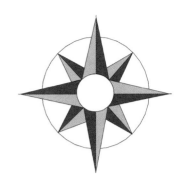

Appendix H.
Annotated Bibliography

A growing number of textbooks have been published on the subject of clinical supervision. Becoming an effective supervisor means learning the theory and practice of clinical supervision, and learning how people learn is a large part of this effort. Practitioners often find it difficult to locate and attend workshops that focus on supervision, so reading about supervision is a good place to begin. Create a lending library at the office or consider joining with a group of colleagues to share what each of you has read. Keep records of all your learning to use for your recertification and professional portfolio. The references listed in this appendix will get you started.

• Bailey, D., & Schwartzberg, S. (2003). *Ethical and legal dilemmas in occupational therapy.* Philadelphia: F. A. Davis.
This excellent text is for those who wish to learn more about common ethical and legal situations that occur frequently in academic and clinical practice. The background information on each situation is articulated clearly, and case studies and commentaries further elucidate the key points.

• Baltimore, M., & Crutchfield, L. (2003). *Clinical supervisor training: An interactive CD-ROM training program for the helping professions.* Boston: Allyn & Bacon.
This cutting-edge technology book contains most of its content on an interactive CD-ROM that permits readers to learn at his or her own pace. More than 65 case vignettes illustrate key concepts of clinical supervision, and each chapter's content is presented in PowerPoint™ lecture format along with recommendations for supplemental reading materials on the basics of clinical supervision. The chapters in the text summarize the content on the CD-ROM and present learning activities. Although this publication is directed toward students in the counseling professions, the case vignettes will permit students to view live supervision sessions, providing rich material for discussion.

• Bernard, J. M., & Goodyear, R. K. (2004). *Fundamentals of clinical supervision* (3rd ed.). Boston: Pearson, Allyn & Bacon.
This classic text, now in its third edition, is a must-read for anyone setting out to provide supervision. Its scope is comprehensive, and its authors are two of the leading researchers in the field of clinical supervision. This text refrains from promoting any single model or method of clinical supervision, providing

readers instead with a broad overview of the field. The authors summarize the relevant research and provide detailed resources for further learning. The book is both scholarly and pragmatic and will be useful to the student learning to supervise and the seasoned practitioner seeking to continue the lifelong learning process. The chapters cover evaluation, models of supervision, ethical and legal considerations, the supervisory relationship, organization of the supervision experience, group and individual supervision, and teaching and researching supervision. The book concludes with a "supervisor's toolbox" containing helpful resources such as sample supervision documents and self-assessments on a variety of topics.

- Brown, G., Esdaile, S., & Ryan, S. (2003). *Becoming an advanced healthcare practitioner.* Philadelphia: Butterworth-Heinemann.

Written by British occupational therapists, this text was one of the first for post-graduate practitioners interested in continuing their learning. The topics presented are not those typically covered in entry-level educational programs and guide readers toward achieving competencies in advanced practice. Although this book does not focus exclusively on clinical supervision, it includes a major chapter on using adult education theories in clinical education.

- Campbell, J. (2000). *Becoming an effective supervisor: A workbook for counselors and psychotherapists.* Philadelphia: Taylor & Francis.

This paperback is presented in an easy-to-follow workbook format. Information is presented concisely at the beginning of each chapter, and extensive exploratory questions follow with space provided for the learner to respond. There are extensive bibliographies at the end of each chapter for further reading, and an appendix contains numerous sample forms. The chapters are functionally oriented, because this text is designed to be practical for students and supervisors alike. The chapters define supervision; identify what supervisors do; describe the models, methods, and techniques of supervision; and address the role of the supervisory relationship, ethical and legal issues, multicultural issues, and administrative tasks. A chapter on the supervisor's personal development addresses important topics such as stress management and ways to avoid burnout.

- Campbell, J. (2006). *Essentials of clinical supervision.* Hoboken, NJ: Wiley.

This pocket-sized paperback is a practical text designed primarily for students and supervisors working in the mental health field. It is written in an easy-to-read style, with key learning points highlighted frequently throughout the book. Each chapter has a short quiz designed to test one's knowledge of the topic just studied before proceeding to the next chapter. The chapters cover models of clinical supervision; formats, methods, and techniques of supervision; ethical and legal issues; and preparations to begin supervising, and three sequential chapters detail the beginning, middle, and advanced stages of supervision. Case examples are presented throughout, as well as sample formats for key supervision documents.

• Costa, D. (2004). *The essential guide to occupational therapy fieldwork education: Resources for today's educators and practitioners.* Bethesda, MD: AOTA Press.
This book is a compendium of documents applicable to fieldwork education, including important AOTA publications related to Level I and Level II fieldwork, policies affecting fieldwork, and resources for fieldwork educators and academic fieldwork coordinators. Practitioners new to supervising fieldwork students or setting up fieldwork programs will find this book very helpful, as will students and experienced fieldwork educators.

• Cross, V., Moore, A., Morris, J., Caladine, L., Hilton, R., & Bristow, H. (2006). *The practice-based educator: A reflective tool for continuing professional development and accreditation.* Hoboken, NJ: Wiley.
This small book was written to provide allied health professionals with a catalyst to continue their professional development and lifelong learning throughout their careers. The book, written by physiotherapists working in the United Kingdom, explores critical themes involved in educating, teaching, mentoring, and supervising the next generation of health care practitioners. It emphasizes the critical role that reflective practice and continuing professional development have in maintaining one's excellence as a health care practitioner. Rather than using terms like *fieldwork educator, clinical instructor,* or *internship coordinator,* which vary across professions, the authors have chosen to use a novel term—*practice-based educator.* Learning outcomes are presented clearly in each chapter with checklists for determining one's own competency and creating a professional development plan. The chapters detail many aspects of clinical education, including adult learning theories. The chapter content is tied into the U.K. health care system but is applicable to practice settings in the United States.

• Falender, C., & Shafranske, E. (2004). *Clinical supervision: A competency-based approach.* Washington, DC: American Psychological Association.
This volume is a comprehensive and scholarly resource designed primarily for psychologists and others supervising mental health practitioners, but it is also useful for professionals from other disciplines providing supervision. Both theory and research are presented in a thorough manner, and competencies for supervisory practice are delineated clearly. Chapters address the practice of good supervision, technical competence, personal factors in supervision, alliance building in supervisory relationships, diversity competence, ethical and legal issues, and evaluation. There is an extensive appendix with sample contracts, self-inventories, multicultural competency assessments, feedback

forms, role conflict and role ambiguity inventories, supervisory competency checklists, and supervisor feedback forms.

• Hawkins, P., & Shohet, R. (2000). *Supervision in the helping professions* (2nd ed.). Philadelphia: Open University Press.

As the title suggests, this book is directed toward all of the helping professions, including occupational therapy. The first two parts of the book address the supervisee's perspective and then the supervisor's perspective. Thus, it appeals both to students in helping them make the most out of supervision and to practitioners as they start to supervise or continue an extensive career. The book addresses a number of personal issues, such as managing stress and avoiding burnout in the helping professions. The authors present their own model of clinical supervision—the double matrix or seven-eyed model of supervision, which they developed in the 1980s. The third and fourth parts of the book address themes such as work with groups and teams in supervision, the organizational context, and training and policy development for clinical supervision. The book concludes with a unique chapter on wounded healers.

• Haynes, R., Corey, G., & Moulton, P. (2003). *Clinical supervision in the helping professions: A practical guide.* Pacific Grove, CA: Brooks/Cole–Thomson Learning.

This book is interactive in approach; suggested learning activities at the end of each chapter help readers integrate the knowledge into their own professional practice. A Web site provides additional learning activities, self-assessments, and resources for further learning. Of particular interest to educators is the companion instructor's manual that contains teaching suggestions, transparency masters, class activities, and a test bank of exam questions. The text features numerous case studies of students and provides questions to facilitate reflection on key concepts. The 11 chapters cover such topics as roles and responsibilities of supervisors, multicultural issues, evaluation, ethical and legal issues in supervision, models and methods of supervision, the supervisory relationship, and ways to become an effective supervisor. The authors are psychologists and counselors with extensive teaching and clinical experience.

• Higgs, J., & Edwards, H. (Eds.). (1999). *Educating beginning practitioners: Challenges for health professional education.* Woburn, MA: Butterworth-Heinemann.

This edited text contains chapters written by some of the leading educators in the United Kingdom and Australia. It is written in a transdisciplinary format and is applicable to students from any health care profession. Some of the chapters focus on classroom teaching, and others focus on clinical teaching; still others focus on increasing students' clinical reasoning skills and teaching research skills and methods.

• Powell, D. (1993). *Clinical supervision in alcohol and drug abuse counseling: Principles, models, methods.* San Francisco: Jossey-Bass.

This is a classic work in the field of clinical supervision, written primarily for practitioners working in the substance abuse field. It presents in detail the author's own blended model of clinical supervision as well as some of the other models of clinical supervision that have been developed. Although most applicable to those working in the specified field, this book provides some interesting historical information on clinical supervision and focuses heavily on the relational issues involved in clinical supervision.

• Privott, C. (1998). *The fieldwork anthology: A classic research and practice collection.* Bethesda, MD: American Occupational Therapy Association.

This is an essential reference for anyone committed to occupational therapy fieldwork education. It is a compendium of classic articles written in peer-reviewed occupational therapy journals since the beginning of the profession in 1917. The collection traces the historical development of fieldwork in the occupational therapy profession. The book also includes research studies on fieldwork outcomes, a good starting point for researchers interested in such questions as what works best, with whom, and in what setting.

• Rose, M., & Best, D. (Eds.). (2005). *Transforming practice through clinical education, professional supervision, and mentoring.* London: Elsevier/Churchill-Livingstone.

This comprehensive text includes the work of contributors from numerous health professions and from the United States, the United Kingdom, Australia, and New Zealand. It addresses the differences between clinical education, professional supervision, and mentoring but unifies the three under their function of transforming professional practice. The book is divided into six sections, with the first four focusing on various aspects and topics in clinical education—learning theories, culture, collaboration, distance learning, evidence-based practice, reflective practice, challenging learning situations, models of clinical education, ethics, and power differential issues. The remaining two sections focus on professional issues such as finding meaning and preventing burnout, obtaining postgraduate clinical supervision, and ways to transform practice. Each chapter has numerous exercises designed to further integrate the reader's knowledge into practice and lists resources for further learning. This book is useful to students and practitioners alike, as well as to academic fieldwork coordinators looking for material to present to occupational therapy fieldwork educators.

• Shepard, K., & Jensen, G. (2002). *Handbook of teaching for physical therapists* (2nd ed.). Boston: Butterworth-Heinemann.

Despite the fact that this text was written for physical therapy educators and practitioners, it contains a wealth of information about the craft of teaching.

Useful chapters discuss patient education, classroom teaching, instructional technology, and clinical education, resulting in a broad level of educational interests. Occupational therapy practitioners will find this book helpful until the occupational therapy profession has a similar text.

• van Ooijen, E. (2003). *Clinical supervision made easy.* Philadelphia: Churchill-Livingstone.

Designed as a brief pocket guide that addresses the practicalities of providing clinical supervision, this text is appropriate for any health care professional providing clinical supervision. It does not specifically address clinical education of students but rather presents summaries of various models of clinical supervision and expands greatly on a model the author has developed, the three-step method of supervision. In Step 1, the focus is on *what:* "What do I need to know?" Step 2 focuses on *how:* "How am I going to find out?" In Step 3, the focus is on *what now:* "What will I do now that I have found out what I wanted to know?"

• Westberg, J., & Jason, H. (1993). *Collaborative clinical education: The foundation of effective health care.* New York: Springer.

The intended audience of this book is any health professional who is now or is planning to begin providing clinical education to students. The content is widely applicable to health care professionals across practice settings. What makes this book unique is its emphasis on the word *collaborative,* and the authors clearly define the differences between a collaborative approach and an authoritarian one, focusing on the process rather than the content of clinical teaching. The four parts of the book each focus on one aspect of the clinical teaching process—thinking about collaborative clinical education, preparing for clinical teaching, doing clinical teaching, and evaluating clinical teaching. Practical suggestions show how to ask questions of learners that facilitate a dialogue and how to develop learning goals and objectives. There is very useful information on the process of giving feedback to others. Each chapter has one or more self-assessments to assist clinical educators in recognizing their own strengths and weaknesses and creating a professional development plan.

See also Recommended Reading.

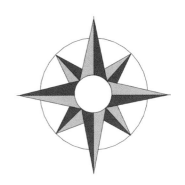

Appendix I.
Guide to the DVD

The enclosed DVD-ROM was created by five of my students who were in the third year of a combined bachelor of science/master of science program. A course from the third year of the curriculum—which focused on instructional methods in teaching—was revamped and presented as a beginning course in clinical supervision. In the new version, students examined some of the content contained in this book: adult learning theories, learning styles, teaching styles, supervision models and theories, and history of fieldwork education in occupational therapy. These five students already had completed two of their three Level II fieldwork experiences, so while they discussed the course topics, they had ample opportunities to reflect on actual situations they encountered in fieldwork.

One of the course assignments had the students create sample supervision scenarios involving fieldwork students. Students were to write scripts for several scenarios that illustrated concepts they discussed in class, such as working with unequal levels of assertiveness skills in students, providing feedback to students, verbal and nonverbal communication skills of the supervisor, designing learning activities for students, and ethical situations. The resulting scripts were the outcomes of their learning, and they alternated roles during filming. The discussion questions are the students' own and may serve to prompt additional questions on the part of the viewer.

This assignment proved to be an excellent learning activity, leading to integration of knowledge with their prior experiences. The scripts they wrote are fictional; no resemblance to actual supervisors or fieldwork settings is intended. The characters in the video, both students and supervisors, are demonstrating less-than-optimal responses, because the intent of this group of students was to be somewhat provocative to facilitate some animated discussion in the viewers.

Viewers are encouraged to watch each scenario in its entirety and then reflect on the questions that follow. Writing a reflective journal activity would be an excellent learning activity for both students and practitioners. Either in groups, dyads, or alone, viewers can rewrite the scenario in a better way, using some of the theories, techniques, and models from this book. This activity will make learning more interactive and active. The narrative outlines and original scripts for each of the five scenarios follow.

Scenario 1

Chrissy is on her third day of a week-long Level I fieldwork in a physical disability setting. She goes along with her supervisor, an occupational therapist, to visit Mrs. Smith.

OT: Good morning Mrs. Smith. This is Chrissy, she is an OT student who is going to be observing and learning from us this morning. Is that OK with you?

Mrs. Smith: Of course, honey. It's nice to meet you. *[They shake hands.]*

OT: Yesterday, during your evaluation, I mentioned that I would be showing you today how to dress your lower body using a hip kit.

Mrs. Smith: Yeah, that sounds great. I had to have the aide dress me this morning.

OT: Before we start, I want to know if you remember your hip precautions.

Mrs. Smith: Alright . . . . the first one is "I can't bend forward," right?

OT: Yup. And . . . ?

Mrs. Smith: Second, "no toes in," and the third . . . hmmmm . . . .

OT: There is one more, can you remember?

Mrs. Smith: No, honey, I can't.

OT: Chrissy, can you tell Mrs. Smith the third precaution?

Chrissy: Mrs. Smith, your third precaution is to never cross your legs.

Mrs. Smith: Oh that's right. Thanks, dear.

OT: Okay, so no toes in, no crossing your legs, and no bending forward.

[Mrs. Smith shakes head in agreement.]

OT: This is called a dressing stick. You are going to use this to help you put on your pants since you can't bend forward.

Mrs. Smith: Oh how wonderful.

OT: First, I'll demonstrate, then, you'll try, so watch carefully.

[OT demonstrates.]

Mrs. Smith: Okay, let me try. *[Tries to do it]* How do I do this again?

OT: Chrissy, do you feel comfortable helping Mrs. Smith?

Chrissy: Okay, as long as you are here watching me.

[END]

Scenario 2

Rebecca has completed 10 weeks of her 12-week Level II fieldwork in an inpatient psychiatric hospital. Jennie has completed 9 weeks of her 12-week Level II fieldwork in the same hospital. Both students have worked closely and have run 3 groups together prior to this one. Jennie has felt throughout the fieldwork that their supervisor has shown favoritism toward Rebecca. Rebecca has tried to ease the situation but is feeling caught in the middle. Rebecca and Jennie just have finished leading a social skills group together while being observed by their occupational therapy supervisor. After every group, the supervisor discusses the outcomes of the group with the students.

OT Supervisor: So . . . what did you think?

Rebecca: I think it went pretty well, I was caught off guard when Joann said, "The only place I like to socialize is at bars," but I think I recovered well.

OT Supervisor: I remember that, it was fine.

[Looks at both students]

Rebecca: Oh . . . and I really liked when Michael participated in the discussion; he is showing a major improvement since Monday.

OT Supervisor: That is a great observation Rebecca . . . . *More silence. Looks at Jennie and stares* AND . . . ?

Jennie: Oh, ummm . . . yeah, I pretty much agree with Rebecca about that and . . . uh . . . well, Mary talked more this group so that's an improvement. *[hopeful smile]*

OT Supervisor: Yeah? I've never known Mary NOT to be a talker. *[Laughs]* Well, anyway I have to go and start my evals for today. I've got three . . . . Oh, but Rebecca you're going to do one for me right? Thanks so much!

[Rebecca nods politely. Supervisor leaves room in a hurry. Rebecca looks uncomfortable.]

Jennie: Why does she hate me so much? *[sits down with her head in her hands]*

[FADE OUT]

Rebecca: Here is the eval I covered for you.

OT Supervisor: Oh, great thanks . . . . What is going on with Jennie?

Rebecca: Why? I thought she did well in group today . . . . She was more vocal than usual . . . . But I think that she's a little intimidated.

OT Supervisor: Ugh, I don't know . . . . I'll figure something out. I wish she was a little more like you. Maybe you can start helping her out.

Rebecca: All right. I'll try.

[END]

Scenario 3

Martha just has completed 7½ weeks of her 12-week Level II fieldwork in an outpatient pediatric clinic. Martha had been treating eight clients a day and completed at least one evaluation every morning prior to treating her clients in the clinic. Her supervisor, Jeanette, just reminded her that she will be treating two more clients everyday and will continue to complete at least three evaluations a week prior to treating in the clinic. Martha already been working from noon to 8 p.m. without taking any breaks during the day. She was starting to feel overwhelmed after her supervisor had informed her of the increased workload and decided to speak with her.

<u>Martha:</u> Jeanette, can I speak with you a minute?

<u>Jeanette:</u> Sure.

<u>Martha:</u> I know that I'm required to treat a full caseload by this time in addition to conducting client evaluations every week, but I'm starting to feel a bit overwhelmed. I feel that I don't have enough time to write up the evaluation reports, treat my clients, and work on my student project.

<u>Jeanette:</u> Well, what would you like me to do?

<u>Martha:</u> I need a half-hour break in between clients to grab some lunch and to finish some paperwork.

<u>Jeanette:</u> Well, in the real world, your supervisor won't give you breaks whenever you need to finish your paperwork. At this point you should be able to treat all your clients without needing a break. You just need to prioritize your time better.

<u>Martha:</u> I am well aware of this, but I'm already doing so much during the day with the evals in the morning and then treating my clients right after—it's too much for me right now.

<u>Jeanette:</u> I'll tell you what—I'll inform the OT director of your request, and I'll let you know what she says.

<u>Martha:</u> Okay.

[LATER THAT DAY]

<u>Jeanette:</u> Martha, I spoke with the director, and she agrees with me. We both think that you should be able to treat all your clients during the day without needing a break. Remember, you have 15 minutes between some clients, and you are aware of the fact that some clients cancel their sessions. You should make good use of that time. Just concentrate on managing your time better.

<u>Martha:</u> I guess so. I'll try to manage my time better.

Jeanette: If anything else comes up, remember that you can always come to me.

Martha: Okay.

[END]

Scenario 4

Level II fieldwork student Cathy is 6 weeks into a 12-week fieldwork in a skilled-nursing facility. Cathy has two supervisors that alternate days. One supervisor works Mondays and Wednesdays, the other works Tuesdays and Thursdays, and Fridays are alternated. Cathy receives a referral for a 75-year-old male patient who fell while at home. Patient is oriented times three but often forgets his way back to his room (which is only two short hallways away), has difficulty remembering to use his walker safely, and often forgets what task he is doing. His daughter claims he fell in the middle of the night because he was confused and unaware of how to safely go to the bathroom.

When filling out an activities of daily living (ADLs) capability list for nursing, Cathy asked her supervisor Diane if this patient should be given an "independent" or "supervision" for toileting. The patient wanted an independent because it meant he could use the bathroom in his room freely and privately without having to ask or wait for nursing. The patient already had begun to use the toilet on his own without telling nursing; consequentially, he had an alarm attached to his wheelchair and clothing to ensure he does not go to the toilet without assistance.

Diane tells Cathy to give the patient an independent for toileting and that she will tell nursing to remove the alarm. Cathy then is questioned by Patti as to why she would give a patient an independent for toileting when he is cognitively limited. Both interactions play out in the video.

Monday

Cathy: Do you have a minute to help me with something?

Diane: Sure, I'm just doing some paperwork.

Cathy: Do you remember the patient I just picked up.

Diane: Yeah, I did his evaluation.

Cathy: Well, nursing has had a hard time keeping him from using the toilet on his own, so he was given a wheelchair alarm to remedy his behaviors. Now I'm filling out his ADL capability sheet for nursing, and I don't know if I should give him an independent or supervision for toileting. He really wants to be able to toilet whenever he has to without having to ask permission, but he does have some cognitive limitations.

Diane: Well, I thought he was able to toilet himself and that he is alert and oriented times three.

Cathy: He is, but his daughter says that he fell at home because he got up to use the bathroom and in his confusion fell.

Diane: Your patient does not have many physical or cognitive limitations. Placing an alarm on him is too much, but I see your concern with toileting. However, I still feel you should give him an independent. As OTs we promote quality of life; it is premature to take away an ADL task that your patient is still capable of doing. His cognition is not so limited that he can't use a toilet in his own room. Please finish your documentation and leave it on my desk.

Tuesday

Patti: I see that you have given your patient an independent for toileting. I thought that he had some cognitive limitations.

Cathy: He does, but they are mild. He really wants to use the toilet on his own and he can, but there are some safety issues.

Patti: Yes, he does have safety issues, and if he falls while he is going to the bathroom, you and I are the ones that become liable for his fall.

Cathy: I realize that it is a liability, but I thought that as OTs we are supposed to promote quality of life for our patients. There are no serious complications with him; he is in therapy because of a fall he had that only resulted in some bruising. Nursing has also placed a wheelchair alarm on him because he refuses to ask to go to the bathroom.

Patti: We can ask nursing to take the alarm off and speak to the patient about the safety and the importance of having a nurse present when he toilets. However, this independent has to be changed from independent to supervision. I understand that you want the best for your patient, but if he falls not only will he have repercussions, so will we.

[END]

Scenario 5

Level II fieldwork student Sarah is 10 weeks into a 12-week physical disabilities placement. Jennifer, a certified occupational therapy assistant (COTA) student, just has begun her first week of rotation at the same site. Sarah's supervisor Barbara decided to create a new challenge for Sarah by having her supervise the COTA student. Sarah does not feel comfortable supervising Jennifer and does not know how she is supposed to supervise.

Barbara: I have a new challenge to help prepare you to be an entry-level therapist.

Sarah: Sure what do you have in mind?

Barbara: I want you to get some experience supervising a COTA, so why don't you supervise Jennifer during her first week while she gets accustomed to this environment. I think it would be a good learning experience for both of you.

Sarah: I'm not sure as to how I'm supposed to supervise. I mean what does Jennifer do when I don't need her help or am I supposed to have her do my work. The COTAs here do their own treatment; I'm not sure what it means to supervise her.

Barbara: Well you could have her do some of your treatment, encourage her to come up with her own activities, and after the first week she'll be getting her own caseload.

Sarah: Did you speak to Jennifer about this? Does she feel comfortable having me supervise her?

Barbara: Don't worry, I'm sure that you will both do fine. You have to be prepared to take on the responsibilities of an occupational therapist, and I think this would be a good exercise.

Sarah: Okay, I guess I'll go supervise.

[END]

Credits

These scenarios and the accompanying DVD-ROM were created by the following graduates of the Class of 2006 of the Occupational Therapy Program at Stony Brook University in New York:

Nella Bastien, MS, OTR/L

Christina Guida, MS, OTR/L

Melissa Jensen, MS, OTR/L

Jamie Sandler, MS, OTR/L

Esther Strusman, MS, OTR/L

Index

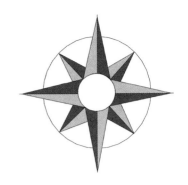

About the Author

Donna M. Costa, MS, OTR/L, is Chairperson of the Occupational Therapy Program at Stony Brook University, New York, and Clinical Associate Professor. She is completing her clinical doctorate in occupational therapy from the University of Indianapolis in 2007 and received a master's degree in health care administration from the New School for Social Research in New York City. She recently has been awarded a large grant to develop at a career laddering program at Stony Brook University for occupational therapy assistants to become occupational therapists. Costa also is serving as the Academic Fieldwork Coordinator Representative on the Commission on Education of the American Occupational Therapy Association and on the Fieldwork Resources Ad Hoc Committee. She is the editor of *The Essential Guide to Fieldwork: Resources for Today's Educators and Practitioners* (AOTA Press, 2004) and has published numerous articles in *OT Practice*. A public speaker and professional trainer on issues related to fieldwork education, complementary and alternative medicine, and a variety of mental health topics, Costa also maintains a clinical practice in mental health, working with individuals with severe mental illness and providing fieldwork supervision to Level I and Level II students.